The Family and Friends' Guide to Diabetes

Everything You Need to Know

Eve Gehling
M.Ed., R.D., C.D.E.

John Wiley & Sons, Inc.

New York • Chichester • Weinheim • Brisbane • Singapore • Toronto

Published by John Wiley & Sons, Inc.
Published simultaneously in Canada

Design and composition by Navta Associates, Inc.

The information contained in this book is not intended to serve as a replacement for professional medical advice. Any use of the information in this book is at the reader's discretion. The author and the publisher specifically disclaim any and all liability arising directly or indirectly from the use or application of any information contained in this book. A health care professional should be consulted regarding your specific situation.

Library of Congress Cataloging-in-Publication Data:
Gehling, Eve
    The family and friends' guide to diabetes : everything you need to know / Eve Gehling.
        p.   cm.
    Includes bibliographical references and index.
    ISBN 0-471-34801-5 (acid-free paper)
    1. Diabetes Popular works. 2. Diabetes—Patients—Family relationships.
I. Title.
RC660.4.G44   2000
616.4'62--dc21   99-39650

Printed in the United States of America
10 9 8 7 6 5 4 3 2 1

Contents

Acknowledgments   v

Note to Readers   vi

Introduction   1

1. Diabetes Facts   5

2. Managing Low Blood Glucose   46

3. Preparing Healthy Meals   72

4. Caring During Illness and High
   Blood Glucose   114

5. Planning Special Occasions with
   Confidence   135

6. Creating Positive Work Environments   154

7. Understanding My Emotions . . .
   to Better Cope with Their Diabetes   190

8. Promoting Healthy Habits at Home   220

9. Building Positive Relationships   237

Appendix A: Suggested Reading List   257

Appendix B: Associations/Agencies to Explore
   and Contact   259

Appendix C: Sample Menus   261

Appendix D: References   263

Index   275

Acknowledgments

I would like to thank all my friends and family (with and without diabetes) who have supported and encouraged me to write this book. Without their ideas and suggestions, this book would not have become a reality as quickly as it did. A special thanks to my husband for his endless support and humor while helping me meet my deadlines. Thank you!!!

Note to Readers

This book is not meant to be used to diagnose or treat medical conditions. It should not be used to replace individual or group education for people with diabetes who would benefit from learning to care for their unique medical needs. This book, instead, is meant to clarify what diabetes is and provide general information on how the disease is treated in order to help friends and family be understanding and supportive to those with diabetes in receiving optimal medical care.

While recognizing that diabetes affects both males and females, the author has attempted to write to both genders in an unbiased fashion. For reading ease and clarity, use of male and female pronouns and names are used interchangeably. If the names and stories used in this book resemble anyone in real life, it is purely coincidental, as names were chosen randomly.

While this book includes examples of food and nonfood items, it is not endorsing any specific products or implying that they are appropriate for use in the diet of every person with diabetes. Those with diabetes should seek the advice of their health care provider, registered dietitian, or certified diabetes educator if they have specific questions about their meal plan.

Introduction

Shocked, George slumped in his chair. His hand still clutching the phone receiver, he sat stunned at the news his mother had just told him—she had diabetes. She had gone to her clinic to get a new pair of glasses only to learn that the cause of her blurred vision wasn't due to her eyes. It was caused by high blood sugar. Although she told him not to worry, that her diabetes wasn't as serious as his cousin Frank's because she only needed to take a pill, he was worried. "How can this be?" he wondered. "Isn't diabetes a serious disease that people die from? How can they diagnose diabetes from an eye exam?"

Susan is frustrated and angry. Her husband has complained she nags him too much about his diabetes. "That's unfair," she fumed. "I wouldn't bug him if I didn't have to worry about him having an insulin reaction. It bothers me when he doesn't eat on schedule, follow his diet, or test his blood glucose levels. He isn't a child—he knows better! But how can I get him to take better care of himself without nagging?"

Betty's perplexed. As an office manager, she celebrates employees' birthdays by bringing in morning treats. Tomorrow is Lisa's birthday. She had planned to bake a cake in Lisa's honor. However, she just remembered that Lisa has diabetes and doesn't usually eat cake or cookies. "What should I do?" she wondered. "If she can't eat cake, there's no reason to bake one. Should I skip bringing in treats tomorrow?"

While the situations above may be different, George, Susan, and Betty all have something in common: They are affected by someone who has diabetes. George is concerned about his mother's health and wonders how diabetes is diagnosed and treated. Susan is unsure of how to cope with her husband's not caring for his diabetes. Betty is unsure how to support a friend and coworker who has a chronic disease. While they all want to help, they are unsure how to do so.

These examples are not uncommon. The emotional, psychosocial, and financial effects diabetes can have upon families can be stressful. Unfortunately, all too often, friends and family members receive little if any education on what diabetes is and how to cope with it. What information they hear is often limited and/or out of date, which causes misconceptions and turns well-intentioned behaviors into disease-management hurdles for the person with diabetes.

This book is a compilation of experiences I have had with diabetes spanning over twenty years. My personal experience with diabetes comes from growing up with a brother, grandparents, friends, and coworkers who have it. Watching how they cope with their condition enabled me to observe firsthand how diabetes can both positively and negatively affect relationships.

As a diabetes educator, nutritionist, and lifestyle behavioral counselor for over ten years, I have been asked countless times by friends and family members of someone with diabetes for advice on what to serve or how to help someone cope with diabetes. Each time I am asked, I'm reminded of how far-reaching the effects of diabetes are. Diabetes can affect everyone—men, women, children, and all ethnic groups. It affects not only the person with it, but potentially everyone—friends, family members, and colleagues—who cares for him or her. Because my colleagues and I wished there was a simple reference book we could refer people to, the idea of this book was born.

If you feel uncertain at times as to how you can help someone cope with diabetes, this book is for you. Written in a question-and-answer format, the chapters are designed to help you learn what diabetes is and how it's treated so that you can become better informed about it. Along the way, helpful tips and facts are included to give practical advice to equip you on how to positively support someone with diabetes.

As you read this book, I hope you know how special you are and how lucky the person with diabetes is to have you in his or her life. Just like a pebble tossed into a lake causes a ripple effect, your efforts to learn how to help someone with diabetes can have a far-reaching impact. Believe in yourself; you can make a difference in the lives of those around you.

CHAPTER 1

Diabetes Facts

YOU'VE GOT WHAT—DIABETES? NO WAY, THAT CAN'T BE TRUE.
ISN'T THAT THE DISEASE WHERE PEOPLE TAKE SHOTS,
CAN'T EAT SUGAR, AND CAN GO BLIND OR LOSE A LEG?

When you first learn that someone you know and care about has diabetes, it's common to feel shocked, afraid, and yet curious—all at the same time. As you try to understand what the disease is, you may feel overwhelmed by questions you'd like answered. You may try to remember what you've heard about diabetes in the past and even call someone (e.g., a relative or a retired nurse who lives on your street) to get the inside story. However, as you find one answer, it may lead to more questions as you realize the impact of what the disease is. Before you know it, you may even wonder how someone's diabetes could affect your relationship with them.

It's normal to have questions about diabetes and want to know what the facts are. Through increasing your knowledge level of the disease, you can help someone with diabetes better cope with the condition. This book is designed to provide you with answers to frequently asked questions on diabetes, and empowering tips on how to become a positive helper.

In this chapter, we will begin by reviewing the nitty-gritty details about the disease—what it is and isn't, who gets it, and how it's treated. It will also point you in the right direction to find more detailed information should you want to continue learning more about diabetes and treatment strategies.

Separating Stories from Fact

If you've talked to others about diabetes, you may have heard varying stories about what life with diabetes is like. While some stories may be sad, others may range from inspiring to downright humorous. If you spoke with friends and family members over the age of forty-five, you may even have heard some horror stories. Older adults can often recall someone they knew when they were growing up—an aunt, cousin, or neighbor—who had diabetes. They may recall the days when people with diabetes used long, thick steel syringe needles that had to be sterilized and hand-sharpened! Some may even remember either the angry-looking red welts that some people with diabetes would develop on their skin where insulin was injected or those who developed complications—kidney failure, foot gangrene, or blindness—and died from diabetes. In times past, having diabetes often meant a shortened life, joblessness, social isolation, and being advised not to dream of going to college or raising a family.

What makes these stories scary is that they are true. However, one needs to remember that these stories are from the past, from a day when diabetes was treated differently. Just as time and technology have changed our lives with computers, satellite television, and microwave ovens, they have also changed how diabetes is treated. Consequently, the outlook of what life with diabetes is and can be like has changed.

Because of research, new medicines, and computers, we are entering a new age of diabetes, an age when the risk of developing diabetes complications can be lower. Just because the word sounds like "DIE-a-betes," people with diabetes can live long, successful lives. People with diabetes today can have a different life ahead of them if they care for their disease.

So don't be scared off by stories you may hear about the old days of diabetes. Instead, learn from them and remember that the good new days of diabetes are dawning. While diabetes is still a serious disease and can't be taken lightly, it can be treated.

Let's start at the beginning, answering simple questions about diabetes.

Q. What is diabetes?

A. Diabetes is a disease in which the body either doesn't make or use insulin properly, which in turn affects the way glucose (sugar) is used for energy. When people have diabetes they might say they have a *"touch of sugar," "high sugar,"* or *"diabetes mellitus."* Whatever they call it, though, it still means they have a problem controlling their blood glucose.

To know what diabetes is, it's important to understand how glucose, insulin, and food relate to each other. Glucose is the fuel that our bodies prefer to run on for energy. It is made from the food we eat and drink. As food is digested in the stomach and intestines, glucose enters the bloodstream to be used by the body cells (muscles and tissues) for energy. However, for the glucose to pass from the bloodstream and into the cells, it needs to pass through a cellular door (called a *receptor site*) that is normally closed. The key that unlocks the door is called *insulin*, a hormone produced by the pancreas that acts like a doorman to open the cellular door and allow glucose to enter the cell. Once in the cell, the glucose is either used for immediate energy or stored for future use as glycogen.

When people have diabetes, their body has difficulty using glucose for energy, as there is something wrong with the way their body makes and/or uses insulin. Either they aren't able to make enough insulin to meet their body's needs, or the way it's working isn't effective. As a result, glucose is not able to enter the cells, which results in the blood glucose level staying higher than normal and the cells running low on energy.

An easy way to understand how glucose works in the body is to picture how gas works in a car. If you've ever driven a car, you know there are two things all drivers must remember about gas.

First, you need to use the right type—unleaded or diesel—in order for the motor to run. Second, you need to keep a certain level of gas in the car's system for it to work. If the gas level goes too low, the car will sputter and stop running. If the gas level is too high, chances are you have added too much gas to the gas tank. While this usually doesn't stop a car from running, the extra gas is wasted because it ends up being spilled over the gas tank and onto the ground.

In the body, glucose acts much like gas in a car. Glucose is the main fuel that the body runs on for energy. The body automatically tries to keep its blood glucose level within the normal range so you'll have the energy you need to feel and work well. However, if the glucose level were to drop below 70 milligrams per deciliter (mg/dl), you would start to feel shaky, lightheaded, or hungry—signals that you're running low on fuel and need to eat food for energy. On the other hand, if after you eat a meal your blood glucose levels stayed above normal, it would signal that glucose isn't getting into your cells for energy. The excess (unused) glucose would spill into your urine to be excreted as your body tried to lower the blood glucose level back to normal.

Without your having to think about it, throughout each day your body's pancreas is hard at work acting like a glucose sensor to regulate and keep your blood glucose level within the normal range. When the pancreas senses that you've eaten food (which raises the glucose level in the blood), it makes and releases insulin into the bloodstream to help the cells use glucose for energy. Conversely, when the glucose levels go below normal, the body releases counterregulatory or stress hormones (e.g., glucagon, epinephrine, cortisol, and growth hormone) to raise the blood glucose levels. What's neat is that you don't have to think about it! Your body is designed to automatically do it for you when you don't have diabetes.

Unfortunately, when people have diabetes, they have to think about how their bodies use glucose for energy. Because their bodies have trouble regulating the blood glucose level, they need to help them out. As with driving a car, instead of having an automatic transmission, they must operate their body like they would drive a manual transmission, helping it out so it can run smoothly.

Q. What is a normal blood glucose level?

A. To work effectively, our bodies try to maintain a certain level (or amount) of glucose circulating in the bloodstream for cells to use as energy. While the level will fluctuate slightly through the course of a day, it usually ranges between 70 and 110 milligrams per deciliter (mg/dl) of blood. In someone who does not have diabetes, a blood glucose level anywhere within this range is considered normal.

When people have diabetes, their bodies have trouble regulating the glucose level within the normal range because of a problem making or using insulin. This results in their glucose level staying high after they eat a meal or snack. In turn, this causes them to feel tired, as their cells are not able to utilize the blood glucose (fuel) they need for energy.

Q. I heard there are different types of diabetes. What are they?

A. While everyone with diabetes shares a common problem (using glucose for energy), there are four different types of diabetes. The four types are type 1, type 2, gestational, and other diabetes. These types vary depending upon what is happening in the body with insulin and glucose. When people are diagnosed with diabetes, their doctor will inform them as to which type they have. But here's how you can quickly tell them apart.

Type 1 Diabetes—This type is the most well known form of diabetes, and affects almost one out of every ten people with diabetes. In the United States, that equals over a half-million people. It used to be called juvenile-onset or insulin-dependent diabetes mellitus (IDDM).

Type 1 affects mostly children and adults under the age of thirty, but can occur at any age. The most common age when people get it is during puberty.

People with type 1 diabetes lose their ability to make insulin. To stay alive, they manually have to do what their pancreas automatically did for them—supply and release insulin into their body to control their blood glucose level. This means they must take insulin shots (injections) every day. If they were to delay taking insulin for too long (varying from hours to days), they could go into a coma and die.

Type 2 Diabetes—This is the most common form of diabetes, affecting nine out of every ten people with diabetes in the United States. Type 2 used to be called adult-onset or non-insulin-dependent diabetes mellitus (NIDDM), or type II diabetes, because it was usually diagnosed in older adults. However, it's starting to be diagnosed in obese teenagers.

Type 2 differs from type 1 in that those with type 2 diabetes are still able to make their own insulin. However, because people with type 2 diabetes are often overweight, they are either no longer making enough insulin (called *insulin deficiency*) or their body isn't using it effectively (called *insulin resistance*). Through healthy eating, exercise, and weight loss, many with type 2 diabetes are able to control their condition without the use of medication. But over time, it's common that many need to use diabetes pills or insulin to help their bodies control their glucose level.

Gestational Diabetes—Gestational diabetes (GDM) is a temporary form of diabetes that appears during the second half of pregnancy. Researchers report that GDM affects 2 to 5 percent of all pregnant women in the United States. Yet, depending upon the population group, the incidence can be much higher. GDM is seen in higher rates in women of African, Hispanic, and Native American backgrounds.

GDM is initially treated with a special diet. If that fails to help control the blood glucose levels, insulin shots may be required. The good news about GDM is that it usually disappears after the baby is born. The bad news is that women who have had GDM are at high risk for developing diabetes later on in life. They may also develop GDM with subsequent pregnancies.

Other—A small number of people may develop diabetes due to other medical conditions or causes. These causes can range from side effects to medications used to treat other medical conditions to pancreatic conditions (e.g., cancer) that affect the pancreas's ability to make insulin.

Maturity-onset diabetes of the young (MODY) is another form of diabetes that occasionally afflicts children and young adults. It's passed down from generation to generation within certain families and can have different forms, each caused by different genetic defects in insulin secretion. People with MODY are treated like those with type 2 diabetes.

> *Did you know . . .*
> *over 90 percent of all the people with diabetes have type 2.*

Q. Is diabetes contagious?

A. Don't worry, diabetes is not contagious. You can't catch it from a friend or family member like you can a cold or the chicken pox. You won't catch it from a kiss or a hug. It's not caused by the food you eat or sitting too close to someone at work or school.

Q. If diabetes isn't contagious, what causes it?

A. So far, no one knows what truly causes diabetes. This puzzles researchers and frustrates those with diabetes who want to know what caused their disease. So far, experts have learned that there are probably different reasons why people get type 1 versus type 2 diabetes. What complicates the puzzle is that diabetes is not just one disease, but a group of diseases that have similar traits and symptoms. Here is what researchers have discovered so far.

What Seems to Cause Type 1 Diabetes

- **Immune Response**—Between 90 and 95 percent of the people with type 1 diabetes seem to experience some type of an autoimmune response that triggers their bodies to make antibodies. These antibodies destroy, accidentally, the beta cells in the pancreas that make insulin, by mistaking the beta cells for a virus that could be harmful to the body. This process doesn't happen overnight—it usually happens gradually over a period of years after the autoimmune response trigger goes off. At first, the remaining beta cells are able to keep up with the body's insulin needs. Nevertheless, over time the remaining cells are also destroyed and the process results in diabetes.

Why does this happen? What triggers the process? Scientists are unsure, but some think it may have something to do with environmental factors, viruses, and genetics. Research is under way to answer these questions.

- **Environment and Viral Factors**—Because people are sometimes diagnosed with type 1 diabetes after a viral illness, scientists wonder if there could be something in our environment that triggers the autoimmune response that destroys the pancreas's beta cells. Studies are looking to see whether certain viruses (e.g., mumps and congenital rubella) could be triggers. Other scientists are looking to see if triggers could include a certain food that we eat or free radicals (atoms with unpaired electrons on them) that are in the air. But don't let this scare you. No clear evidence exists as to the role environmental factors may play in causing diabetes or whether they are just interesting coincidences.

- **Genetics**—Diabetes sometimes occurs more often in some families than in others. Because of this, health experts have been searching for genetic (inherited) causes. Through studying cellular DNA—the building and operating codes within cells—several genes have been identified as possibly being protective against or promoting diabetes. One type of gene that may play a role in promoting type 1 diabetes is the human leukocyte antigen (HLA). Children who have certain HLA genes have been found to develop type 1 diabetes at much higher rates than children who do not have them. However, more needs to be learned about the different types of HLA genes to fully understand their role and determine how doctors can practically use genetic information in the treatment and possible prevention of diabetes.

- **Unknown Reasons**—A confusing piece to the puzzle of what causes diabetes is that some people get type 1 diabetes for no logical reason. Some people develop type 1 diabetes without having a family history of diabetes, without antibodies or HLA genes, and despite living a healthy lifestyle. While the number of people affected this way is small, it seems to happen more often in people with African or Asian ethnic backgrounds. When diabetes happens for no known reason, it's called *idiopathic diabetes*.

What Seems to Cause Type 2 Diabetes

- **Age and Genetics**—As people age, their risk level for diabetes increases. Having a family history of diabetes also seems to play a role in developing type 2 diabetes. Experts know that people with Native American, African, Asian, Hispanic, and Pacific Island backgrounds are at higher risk for developing type 2 diabetes than those of Caucasian background.

  However, the link between HLA genes and type 2 diabetes is not clear as it is with type 1 diabetes. So far, it appears that there may be different genes that promote type 2 diabetes than with type 1. A biochemical defect may also play a role.

- **Lifestyle and Obesity**—It's estimated that 80–90 percent of those with type 2 diabetes and who have a family history of diabetes are overweight. Lifestyle habits that can promote weight gain (e.g., eating a diet high in excess calories and fat and being inactive) can increase one's risk for developing diabetes. Having extra body fat, especially around the abdominal area (stomach fat versus fat that collects mostly on the hips), can sometimes lead to insulin resistance. This can make it harder for the body to control its blood glucose level.

- **Environmental Factors**—The environment one lives in appears to play a role in developing type 2 diabetes. Countries and cultures that adopt a "western lifestyle" are experiencing increasing rates of diabetes. This is thought to be due to eating a higher fat, lower complex carbohydrate diet, having a lower (or sedentary) activity level, and obesity.

What Seems to Cause Gestational Diabetes

Just as the causes of type 1 and 2 diabetes are unknown, so is the cause of gestational diabetes. We know that during pregnancy a woman's blood glucose control worsens in the last trimester or three months. Health experts believe this may be caused by hormone and weight changes that naturally occur with pregnancy. Usually, a woman's pancreas is able to compensate by producing extra insulin. However, some women's bodies are unable to keep up, which results in their blood glucose levels staying elevated. These women develop gestational diabetes.

Because nearly 40 percent of women who have gestational diabetes develop type 2 diabetes later in life, the role that genetics, lifestyle, and obesity play as causal agents is being studied.

What Seems to Cause the Other Remaining Types of Diabetes

Did you know . . . diabetes is not contagious or caused by the food someone eats.

Diabetes and high blood glucose levels can result from other medical conditions and treatments. Here are some examples of what can cause diabetes symptoms:

- pancreatic disorders (e.g., pancreatic cancer, chronic pancreatitis, cystic fibrosis)

- genetic disorders (e.g., Down and Turner's syndrome)

- polycystic ovary syndrome

- infections (e.g., congenital rubella)

- endocrine disorders (e.g., Cushing's syndrome and hyperthyroidism)

- some drugs (e.g., steroids and nicotinic acid)

Q. How does a doctor know when someone has diabetes? How is it diagnosed?

A. Years ago, doctors used to diagnose diabetes using urine tests. However, because urine tests only showed the amount of glucose that spilled into the urine as the kidneys tried to cope with high blood glucose levels, the tests were not precise. Today, doctors diagnose diabetes with the help of blood tests that are much more accurate.

There are two common blood tests that can be performed in a doctor's office to diagnose diabetes—a blood (plasma) glucose test and an oral glucose tolerance test. The quickest is the blood glucose test, which consists of taking a small blood sample (usually from the arm) and having it tested in a lab to see how much glucose is present. This test can be done either randomly or after fasting. A random blood glucose test can be taken at any given time during the day. In contrast, a fasting blood glucose test requires that no food be eaten for at least eight hours before the test is taken. A fasting test is most commonly done early in the morning, before eating breakfast.

The oral glucose tolerance test (OGTT) takes a little longer to do, as it consists of drinking a liquid containing 75 grams of glucose (50 or 100 grams for pregnant women) and then doing blood glucose tests. Blood samples are taken before drinking the liquid and afterwards at thirty-minute, one-hour, two-hour, and three-hour intervals. The OGTT assesses how quickly a person's body is able to return its blood glucose level back to normal after ingesting glucose.

If any of the tests reveal that the glucose level is above normal, the doctor will retest the level on another occasion. A diagnosis of diabetes is made, then, based on having two elevated blood glucose readings in any of the following three ways:

- a fasting plasma glucose level greater than or equal to 126 mg/dl (or 7.0 millimoles per liter—mmol/L)
- a random plasma glucose level greater than 200 mg/dl (11.1 mmol/L) and symptoms of diabetes

- a two-hour OGTT glucose level greater than 200 mg/dl (11.1 mmol/L)

A diagnosis of gestational diabetes is made when a pregnant woman has any two of the following results:

- a fasting plasma glucose level greater than or equal to 105 mg/dl (5.8 mmol/L)

- an OGTT plasma glucose level greater than 190 mg/dl (10.6 mmol/L) after one hour, greater than 165 mg/dl (9.2 mmol/L) after two hours, or greater than 145 mg/dl (8.1 mmol/L) after three hours

---

Did you know . . . in some countries doctors measure glucose levels in millimoles per liter (mmol/L) instead of milligrams per deciliter (mg/dl). To convert from one unit of measure to the other, use this formula.

mmol/L = mg/dl ÷ 18 (e.g., 7.0 mmol/L = 126 mg/dl ÷ 18)
mg/dl = mmol/L × 18 (e.g., 126 mg/dl = 7.0 mmol/L × 18)

Q. My father-in-law says he has "borderline diabetes." What does this mean?

A. The term "borderline diabetes" is misleading. Sometimes when people first hear this term they picture someone teetering or standing in the middle of a doorway—literally standing on the edge of a border. The person can see what's ahead in the next room, but hasn't crossed over the border yet. And if they had their choice, they would never cross, as doing so would mean they have a disease—diabetes. However, if they stay on the border, some believe they are safe from health problems. That is the misleading part, and here's why.

Prior to 1997, diabetes was diagnosed when someone had a fasting blood glucose level over 140 mg/dl. The difference within this level and 110 mg/dl (what is considered the highest normal blood glucose level) created a thirty-point gap (border) between having a normal glucose level and being diagnosed with diabetes. When someone's blood glucose level consistently stayed within the 110-to-140 mg/dl range, they were told they had "borderline diabetes" or a "touch of sugar." While they did not have diabetes yet, it meant they were close to having it.

So what was misleading about the term "borderline diabetes"? Well, many people believed that as long as they had

> **Did you know . . . years ago, doctors used to diagnose diabetes by testing people's urine. If the urine felt sticky, tasted sweet, and smelled like honey, it was a positive sign that they were spilling glucose into their urine and had diabetes.**

not crossed the "border" yet, they were fine. Some decided to wait until their doctor told them they had crossed the border before learning about diabetes and how to prevent or delay it. Many didn't see their doctor for annual checkups, which resulted in their glucose level not being monitored on a regular basis. By putting off checkups and choosing to wait and see what developed, they didn't take their rising glucose level seriously.

It's unfortunate, but many people don't realize that diabetes develops slowly and can quietly creep up on someone over time. By the time people are diagnosed with type 2 diabetes, over half already have started developing health-related problems (eye, blood pressure, or heart problems). If people took "borderline diabetes" more seriously, they could take steps to preserve their health by delaying or even preventing the onset of diabetes.

In 1997, the American Diabetes Association (ADA) took action to encourage those people with elevated glucose levels and at risk for developing type 2 diabetes to take steps to stay healthy. Here's what they did.

First, they dropped the fasting blood glucose level used to diagnose diabetes from 140 mg/dl to 126 mg/dl. This reduced the gap in half (making it only 15 points) between having normal glucose levels and diabetes. Through earlier diagnosis and treatment of diabetes, experts hope to prevent and/or delay many of the harmful health complications people with diabetes have suffered from in the past.

Second, they recommended that instead of using the term

"borderline diabetes," health care professionals use the term "glucose impairment," as it better explains what's happening in the body, and urge those with it to take earlier action to learn about diabetes. There are two types of glucose impairments people may be told they have, based upon how their glucose level was tested. They may have impaired fasting glucose or impaired glucose tolerance.

Impaired Fasting Glucose (IFG): This term describes someone who has a fasting blood glucose level between 110–126 mg/dl. It means that their glucose is above normal (greater than 110mg/dl) but not high enough to be diagnosed with diabetes (less than 126 mg/dl).

Impaired Glucose Tolerance (IGT): This term describes someone who has taken an oral glucose tolerance test and had a two-hour blood (plasma) glucose level of 140–200 mg/dl.

Currently, it's estimated that 21 million Americans have impaired glucose tolerance, of which 35–40 percent will later go on to develop type 2 diabetes. Because of this high risk, those diagnosed with a glucose impairment should consider their diagnosis a serious health concern and start taking measures to decrease their risk for developing diabetes in the future. These measures might include making changes in their lifestyle habits to eat healthier, be more physically active, maintain a desirable weight level, and reduce or manage their stress level. In addition, they should have their blood glucose level checked on a regular basis.

> **How can I help?**
> If you know someone who has a glucose impairment, encourage him or her to lead a healthy lifestyle to reduce their risk of diabetes.

Q. What symptoms do people have when they get diabetes?

A. While the symptoms of diabetes can vary slightly from person to person, it's easy to recognize them once you know how they relate to each other and to how the body reacts to having a high glucose level.

What Happens in the Body	→	Symptoms
When glucose levels are high, the body tries to excrete the extra glucose in the urine, causing a frequent need to go to the bathroom.		Increased urination
Because they're urinating a lot, people feel unusually thirsty.		Increased thirst
Because the cells aren't getting glucose for energy, they signal the body to eat (take in food for glucose).		Increased hunger
Because cells aren't getting glucose for energy, they start to feel tired and weak.		Fatigue, unexplained weight loss
High glucose levels affect the eyes.		Blurred vision
High glucose levels start to affect the white blood cells' ability to fight infection.		Poor healing wounds, recurring skin, gum, or bladder infections

When blood glucose levels remain high (over 250 mg/dl) for too long (over weeks to years), a person may begin to feel additional symptoms that require prompt medical treatment:

- weakness
- dehydration
- dry mouth
- low blood pressure
- difficulty breathing
- fruity odor on breath
- shock
- coma

Q. How is diabetes treated?

A. The cornerstone of all diabetes treatment is healthy lifestyle habits—eating nutritious meals and being physically active. Education on the use of medications, regular monitoring of glucose levels, and self-care management are individually prescribed to meet the unique needs of each person.

Healthful Eating
People with diabetes are advised to follow a meal plan that helps them space their food intake out throughout each day. This helps to keep the amount and type of food eaten consistent,

which in turn helps them to stabilize their glucose level and maintain a desirable weight. Chapter 3 will explain more about how the diet works.

Lifestyle Habits

Leading a healthy lifestyle includes being physically active, exercising on a regular basis, and managing stress. Regular physical activity can increase insulin sensitivity in the body and lower blood glucose levels. It can also help relieve stress, support efforts to not gain weight, and promote a sense of general well-being. For those with type 2 diabetes, modest weight loss can also help manage diabetes.

Blood Testing

Diabetes treatment includes routine blood glucose checks, at home and at the doctor's office. At home, people are taught to do self-monitoring using portable glucose meters.

Medication

People with type 1 diabetes need to take insulin, as their bodies are no longer able to make it. People with type 2 diabetes may need to take a diabetes pill and/or insulin, depending upon what their bodies need. There are a number of diabetes pills that may be used alone or in combination with each other.

Did you know . . . diabetes is not a new disease. While it's been around for thousands of years, it wasn't until the early 1920s that an effective treatment was discovered, called insulin.

Q. How do the diabetes pills work?

A. Currently, there are four types of diabetes pills used to treat diabetes in the United States. The first type are called *sulfonylureas* (e.g., glimepiride, glipizide, glyburide, chlorpropamide, and tolbutamide) and lower blood glucose levels by helping the pancreas produce more insulin. The second type are called *biguanides* (e.g., metformin) and help lower blood glucose levels by making the liver cells more sensitive to insulin, which results in their making less glucose from stored energy. The third type are α-glucosidase inhibitors (e.g., acarbose), which lower blood glucose levels by working in the intestinal tract to interfere with complex carbohydrates breaking down into glucose. The fourth type are *glitazones* (e.g., rosiglitazone and troglitazone), which lower blood glucose levels by helping the muscle cells become more sensitive (less resistant) to insulin and decreasing the amount of glucose the liver cells make by making the liver cells more sensitive to insulin also.

Q. Where does insulin come from?

A. Two Canadians, Frederick Banting and Charles Best of the University of Toronto, discovered insulin in the early 1920s. By studying the pancreases of dogs, they successfully learned how to extract insulin from animal pancreases, suspend it in a solution, and inject into a dog to treat its diabetes. The dog did not die from its diabetes! Next, they found ways to extract insulin from cow and pig pancreases, which could be used to treat humans with diabetes. Although the early insulin solutions created weren't perfect, they were close enough and ever since have saved the lives of millions of people and animals.

After years of study, in the 1970s scientists established a way to purify insulin made from animal sources so humans using it experienced fewer side effects. Up until then, sometimes people with diabetes were sensitive to the animal insulin and would develop thick, pitted skin where the insulin was repeatedly injected. Some had allergic reactions that caused rashes or red welts on their skin. For those who experienced these problems, purified insulins offered them relief from unpleasant side effects.

In the 1980s and 1990s, research took insulin manufacturing a giant step forward as a process was created to make synthetic human insulin from *E. coli* bacteria. Called human insulin, because it was a near-perfect match to the kind of insulin the human body makes, it caused few side effects and could be produced from nonanimal sources. Today, synthetic human insulin is the insulin of choice for people with diabetes.

Q. My brother uses a type of insulin that he says is super-fast. What is this type of insulin and what does he mean by "fast"? What does insulin look like?

A. There are five basic types of insulin that people use for injections: quick, short, intermediate, long, and combination acting. These are based on how fast they work. Quick or fast acting insulin (Lispro) starts to work within fifteen minutes of taking it. Because it works so quickly, people who use it need to eat their meals right after they take it—they shouldn't delay eating; otherwise they run the risk of having a low blood glucose level. Short acting insulin (regular) takes a little longer (30 minutes) to start working. People who use regular insulin usually inject it a half-hour before they eat. This insures that the insulin will be most effective to control their blood glucose level when their body is digesting their meal.

Intermediate and long acting insulins, on the other hand, work more slowly than quick and short acting insulin. This is because they contain chemicals that delay their action so they can be taken just once or twice a day, in comparison to the faster insulins, which are taken two to four times per day.

Insulin Type	Name	Starts Working In:	Most Effectively Working In:
Rapid	Lispro	15–30 min	30–90 min
Short	Regular	30–60 min	2–4 hours
Intermediate	NPH	2–4 hours	6–10 hours
	Lente	3–4 hours	4–12 hours
Long	Ultralente	6–12 hours	10–16 hours

Insulin is usually packaged as a liquid in either a glass vial or cartridge. Quick acting insulin is clear in color, while longer acting insulin looks cloudy (milky), as it has chemicals added that delay how fast it works. Insulin that is sealed (unopened) is best stored in a refrigerator until it's used or reaches its expiration date. Once a vial or cartridge is opened, the insulin remains good for one month if it's kept at room temperature.

Did you know . . .
the amount of insulin someone takes doesn't mean his or her diabetes is better or worse than someone else's; it just means the body's insulin needs are different.

Typically, people taking insulin to treat their diabetes take one to four injections a day, depending upon which type of insulin is used and what their body needs are. Unless one is using an insulin pump or special air-pressured injector, injections are given using a fine-needle syringe. If two different types of insulin are used, they can be drawn up into the same syringe so only one shot has to be taken. Insulin absorption is best when it's injected into the layer of fatty tissue beneath the skin of the abdomen. However, the arms, legs, and buttocks are often used as alternative injection sites.

For convenience, manufacturers mix short acting and intermediate insulin together to form combination insulin, which has the dual action of the insulins mixed. Because combination insulin is premixed, it is a handy product for people with poor eyesight to use, as it makes drawing up insulin from a vial into a syringe easier.

Q. What is the best type of insulin for people to use?

A. While all insulin is effective in lowering blood glucose levels, the type used should be matched up to the unique needs of each person. Doctors prescribe different types and combinations of insulin depending upon a person's needs and lifestyle. The amount of insulin that a person needs is based upon their body size and sensitivity to insulin. While some people may need to take only small doses of insulin, others need larger ones. The amount of insulin someone needs doesn't mean his or her diabetes is milder or worse than someone else's. Just as every person is different, so are their insulin needs. Their need may even change over time, so they may not use the same dose or insulin type throughout their entire life.

Q. Why can't insulin be taken as a pill? Why does it need to be injected?

A. Insulin is a hormone that is made out of amino acids, like the protein in meat. If you were to swallow insulin, your stomach would chemically digest it, like meat. If this happens, it will no longer work. To be effective, insulin needs to get into the blood-stream intact (whole). For now, the easiest way to do that is to inject the insulin into the fatty tissue underneath the skin where it can directly enter the bloodstream.

Scientists are testing new ways people can take insulin in the future that doesn't require injecting it into the skin with syringes. Three ways being studied include: implantable insulin pumps, insulin patches for the skin, and nasal sprays using insulin powder that can be inhaled through the lungs.

Q. What are finger-stick blood glucose tests?

A. A finger-stick blood glucose test is a test people with diabetes can do themselves using a portable glucose meter. Finger-stick tests consist of pricking one's finger with a lancet (small needle or razor) and placing a small drop of blood on a special test strip, which is inserted into a small meter. In less than a minute, the meter is able to measure and report back how much glucose is in the blood.

Because the meter is small—many are smaller than a deck of cards—finger-stick tests can be done almost anywhere—at home, work, school, or even on an airplane. This convenience allows people the ability to test their blood glucose level on a daily basis. Depending upon what their diabetes treatment program is, some may check several times a day.

By keeping track of their blood glucose readings, people with diabetes are able to manage their diabetes better. For most people, doctors will prescribe a blood glucose goal before meals somewhere between 80 and 140 mg/dl. This goal is like a target or a bull's-eye that they are aiming for. Some days they may have blood glucose readings that are right on target; other times, they may be slightly higher or lower. Variance is normal and expected. However, when blood glucose levels remain consistently out of the target range, the person with diabetes needs to examine his or her diabetes treatment program to determine what is affecting their control.

People with medical conditions in addition to their diabetes may have slightly different target blood glucose goals. During pregnancy, women with diabetes may strive to achieve a tighter or more near-normal goal of 60–100 mg/dl to help promote a healthy pregnancy. Those people who have conditions like kidney or heart disease or are older may be prescribed a slightly higher target blood glucose goal, ranging somewhere between 100 and 200 mg/dl.

An alternative to finger-stick blood tests is to use a battery-operated laser meter where a person inserts a finger into a portable device that uses a powerful beam of light (laser) to vaporize a tiny hole in the finger and measure the body's glucose level. While still being perfected, this is potentially a less painful way to test one's glucose level than pricking one's finger with a lancet. However, because the technology is still new, it is currently more expensive than the traditional meters.

Another alternative to finger-stick blood tests is a portable meter that takes a small blood sample from body areas other than the fingers. While this still requires "poking," it allows a person to obtain a blood sample from areas such as the arm or leg that aren't as sensitive as fingers. This is popular with people who use their fingertips for typing or to play musical instruments. Researchers are inventing new ways to measure blood glucose levels that don't rely on blood samples—these should become available in the new millennium.

Q. My mother used to say that she had brittle diabetes. What does that mean?

A. Diabetes used to be called brittle when it was very hard to control. For little or no reason, the glucose level would seem to swing either high or low. It was frustrating for the person with diabetes, as he or she never knew what to expect or how to plan ahead to prevent it.

Calling someone's diabetes brittle changed, though, when self-monitoring blood glucose (SMBG) meters became available in the 1980s. SMBG meters allowed people to do finger-stick blood glucose checks at home whenever and wherever they wanted to. They didn't have to go to their doctor's office for a plasma blood glucose test, which was often done only once or twice a year. Through daily blood glucose monitoring, people were able to track their glucose levels accurately and learn to make adjustments in their medication, insulin, diet, or exercise level to correct highs and lows.

Consequently, the term "brittle diabetes" is rarely used anymore since glucose levels can be well controlled, in most cases, through education, medications, and self-monitoring.

Q. My wife's blood glucose level fluctuates a lot. Sometimes it's fine and then—poof—it's high for no reason that we can figure out. What can cause glucose levels to rise?

A. There are many factors that can cause blood glucose levels to rise, including food, medications, and illness. When interpreting blood glucose readings, look for patterns. If you see numbers that are way out of her target range— whether high or low—consider if any of the factors listed in the table on page 27 could have contributed to the reading.

By tracking blood glucose levels routinely with a meter, you can look for patterns to help figure out what's going on with her diabetes. If your wife has an occasional blood glucose reading that is high for no reason, don't panic. Sometimes this happens for no apparent reason and should be expected. For people who take insulin to manage their diabetes, it's nearly impossible to have readings that are always perfectly in range.

The next time your wife has an unusually high glucose reading, start watching to see if she develops a pattern of higher readings on three or more occasions after certain events happen. See if you can pinpoint a possible cause for the reading. For example, if she has higher glucose readings on the days she eats out at a certain restaurant, start exploring if there is a relationship between what she's eating there and what the reading is. However, if she is at home eating the same foods and doing her normal activities, but notices higher glucose readings after starting a new blood pressure medication, she should discuss this pattern with her doctor. Her doctor may adjust her medications to help correct the problem.

By learning to watch blood glucose patterns, you'll feel more in control of what's happening with your wife's diabetes because you'll learn what can affect her glucose level both negatively and positively. Through watching patterns, your wife will be able to plan ahead or take steps to adjust her diet, activity level, or insulin for times when you expect her glucose level to go higher or lower. This is called *diabetes pattern management.* If your wife doesn't know how to do this or you'd like to learn more about pattern management, work with her diabetes educator or health provider to learn how to do so.

Did you know . . . controlling diabetes is like juggling tennis balls. There are many things— diet, exercise, medications, illness, and stress—that can cause the glucose level to get out of control. But with practice, it gets easier.

Factors That Affect Blood Glucose Levels	Possible Blood Glucose Level Effect
Food (type and amount)	↑ or ↓ glucose levels

Beverages:
  Alcohol
  Sweetened drinks
	↓ glucose levels
	↑ glucose levels

Activity level	↑ or ↓ glucose levels
Medications	↑ or ↓ glucose levels
Poor health (illness, trauma, infection, or surgery)	↑ glucose levels
Menstrual cycle (for women)	↑ glucose levels

Q If someone has to take three or four shots of insulin a day, their diabetes must be pretty bad, right?

A. The number of insulin shots someone needs to take during a day does not indicate how good or bad someone's diabetes is. (Only blood glucose tests can tell how well someone's diabetes is controlled.) However, the number of insulin shots someone takes can give you a clue as to the type of insulin program they use and how aggressively they're managing their diabetes.

There are two types of insulin therapy used to treat diabetes: conventional and intensive. Conventional therapy consists of taking one or two shots of insulin a day. This is the most common insulin therapy program used by people with types 1 and 2 diabetes. Intensive therapy, on the other hand, tailors the type and dose of insulin used to the unique needs of those with diabetes. With this program, people strive to control their blood glucose levels more tightly while at the same time allowing for more flexibility in their meals and schedules. While more flexibility with what can be eaten and when sounds great, intensive therapy programs aren't for everyone, as they consist of taking three to four insulin shots per day or using an insulin pump. It also requires frequent (at least 4 times per day) blood glucose testing. Not everyone is motivated enough to do this. For those who are, though, it can provide a greater feeling of control over their diabetes.

> *How can I help? If you find out that someone with diabetes uses an intensive insulin program to control, commend him or her on the hard work they do to keep their blood glucose level in control.*

Q. My son is thinking about getting an insulin pump. What's a pump?

A. An insulin pump is a device people with diabetes can use to supply a steady stream of insulin to their body in a way that mimics what their pancreas used to do. It's an option for those who need to use insulin, want tighter glucose control with fewer highs and lows, and need greater flexibility with their meal plan and schedules.

While the pump is a small, square device that looks like a personal pager or the portable radio walkers or runners use, it is really a tiny computer that holds enough insulin to last a few days. The pump can be either clipped onto a person's belt like a pager or kept in a pocket, close to the body. Attached to the pump is a small piece of tubing that has a needle on its end. The pump user inserts the needle under their skin and tapes it down so it doesn't move. The pump is then programmed to release a steady stream of insulin into the body, day and night. When the user eats a meal or snack, they can program the pump to deliver extra insulin (called a *bolus*). Pumps are mainly used by people with type 1 diabetes who need to take insulin every day.

Q. Why doesn't everyone taking insulin use a pump?

A. That's a question that has many answers, because there are pros and cons to using pumps. The benefits to using a pump are that it often allows users to achieve tighter control over their blood glucose level. Pumps allow for more flexibility with meals and schedules, which is helpful to those people who lead active lives or hold jobs that demand flexible schedules. People who use pumps often report that they enjoy the pumps, as they don't have to worry about carrying syringes and taking shots anymore. On the downside, though, pumps are expensive to buy and maintain if they are not covered under someone's medical insurance policy. Not everyone can afford to use them. In addition, using a pump means that someone doesn't mind being attached to it all the time (even when sleeping!). Pump users also need to be willing to test their blood glucose levels at least four to six times a day. They need to take precautions so that they don't develop infections where the needle is inserted. They also need to receive special training on how to care for their pumps so that they know what to do if the pump fails, which can happen if the battery runs low or the tubing becomes clogged. Because of this, many with diabetes prefer not to use a pump.

Q. My husband's aunt says she has a mild case of diabetes that doesn't require that she use diabetes pills or insulin. What does this mean?

A. Just as Shakespeare wrote, "What's in a name? that which we call a rose/By any other name would smell as sweet," diabetes is still diabetes, no matter how it's described. Either someone has it or they don't. It's kind of like being pregnant—either you are or you aren't. There are no in-between stages.

Some health care providers and people casually use the word "mild" to describe a person with type 2 diabetes who is able to control the disease through weight control, healthy eating, and physical activity. However, this term is rather misleading, as it insinuates that if someone has "mild diabetes," then someone else could have a different (opposite) form of diabetes that's "severe or vicious." By using the word "mild" to describe diabetes, it can sometimes lead people to think that their diabetes isn't bad. But the fact is clear: Diabetes is a serious, chronic disease, no matter which type someone has. Having diabetes should not be taken lightly by either persons with it or their friends and family members.

A concern that exists with describing type 2 diabetes as a mild or less serious form of the disease is that it can result in some people not paying close attention to their diabetes treatment program. Because they don't need to take insulin, they can become lax in doing self-care management and testing their blood glucose level on a regular basis. They may accept suboptimal blood glucose levels so that they don't have to take pills or insulin, which would imply, to their misunderstanding, that their diabetes was now worse or more severe. No one wants to have a severe disease if they have a chance to have a mild one.

So instead of calling diabetes "mild," it would be better if everyone simply called diabetes what it is—diabetes. This could help people with and without diabetes better understand that diabetes is treated in different ways and that people who need to use insulin or pills to regulate their blood glucose level aren't worse off than people who don't need to; their diabetes is just treated differently, to reflect their unique needs.

Q. My husband was diagnosed with type 2 diabetes five years ago and initially had to take pills to control his glucose. But after losing twenty pounds, he no longer has to take pills. He says that his diabetes has gone away and he's cured. Is he right?

A. Unfortunately, there's no cure for diabetes. Once someone has it, they always have it. After making initial lifestyle changes (eating healthier, becoming active, and losing weight) and starting to use diabetes pills or insulin, some people think that their diabetes has gone away. This is because their blood glucose level may improve to a point where they no longer need medication. This is what happened with your husband.

Because your husband made healthy lifestyle changes and is no longer overweight, he is able to manage his diabetes without the use of medications. But his diabetes hasn't gone away—he's just able to treat it differently. He needs to remember that his diet and activity plan is his prescribed treatment for diabetes and is just as important as taking pills or insulin. If your husband were to regain his weight by not watching his diet and becoming less active, he would run the risk that his blood glucose control could worsen. He could need medication again.

In people with type 1 diabetes, after starting insulin treatment some people may think that their diabetes has gone away because their glucose control improves temporarily to a point where they need very little or no insulin injections. This temporary diabetes remission (called the *honeymoon phase*) can last for a number of months. The honeymoon phase happens after the initial insulin treatment returns the glucose levels to normal, which enables the few remaining pancreas beta cells that make insulin to temporarily recover and make enough insulin to meet their body's needs. However, over time, these remaining cells are destroyed from the autoimmune response (like the previous ones were), and the person needs to restart taking insulin to compensate.

Q. My sister got diabetes right after Halloween, when she ate a lot of candy. Does eating too much sugar cause diabetes?

A. Over the years, there have been many diabetes questions that people wonder about. Often the answer is limited to how much is known about diabetes at the time the question is asked.

Did you know . . . if someone with type 2 diabetes needs to start taking insulin, it doesn't mean that they've failed—it just means their body needs more insulin than it can make.

Over the past hundred years, though, we've learned a lot about diabetes. Unfortunately, not everyone has the updated facts. Because people often learn about diabetes from friends or family members, sometimes what gets shared aren't the updated facts. This results in horror stories and myths being passed around.

But not anymore. It's time to set the record straight and share the news about what we know about diabetes today. Here are the top 7 diabetes myths that need to be laid to rest.

Myth #1: Eating too much holiday sweets or candy causes diabetes.

Fact: Eating sugar or sweets does not cause diabetes. If it did, everyone who eats candy and cookies would have diabetes.

It's easy to understand how this myth started. For years, people with diabetes have been told to avoid sugar and sweets, as it would raise their blood glucose (sugar) level. Thus, there is an association between diabetes and eating sugar. However, this association is a problem only for people who already have diabetes because their bodies are unable to effectively use glucose for energy—not sucrose (table sugar). People without diabetes are able to make plenty of insulin and control their glucose level.

Another reason why eating too much holiday candy or sugar doesn't cause diabetes is that diabetes doesn't usually happen overnight. Instead, it develops gradually. Research shows that diabetes can start developing almost ten years before the onset of type 1 diabetes. For type 2 diabetes, the average is six to seven years.

What is true about sugar is that eating too much of it can lead to an intake of too many calories. Eating more calories than a body needs leads to weight gain. Being overweight, in turn, increases a person's risk for developing type 2 diabetes if they have a family history of diabetes and other risk factors for diabetes (see page 44). Consequentially, eating too many sweets can indirectly increase one's risk for diabetes; however, sweets by themselves do not cause diabetes.

Myth #2: Everyone with diabetes takes insulin shots.

Fact: Of all the people with diabetes, less than half need to treat their disease with insulin shots. While it's true that everyone with type 1 diabetes needs to take insulin, only 40 percent of those with type 2 diabetes need to, as most are able to make some of their own insulin. That leaves roughly 9 million people (60% of people with type 2 diabetes) who are able to manage their disease through a combination of diet, exercise, and/or diabetes pills. That many people prove this myth to be false.

Myth #3: Insulin shots hurt.

Fact: Twenty to thirty years ago, insulin shots did hurt, because the needles used were thick and needed to be hand-sharpened when they got dull. However, those are the needles of the past. Today, syringe needles are disposable, so they are always sharp. They are also so thin that a mosquito bite hurts worse. Many people don't even feel the needles going into their skin. Ask anyone who takes insulin shots and they'll tell you—insulin shots aren't hard once you get used to giving them. Pricking their fingers to test their blood glucose level is what they would rather not have to do.

Myth #4: If you use insulin to treat your diabetes, you'll go blind.

Fact: Insulin doesn't cause blindness—diabetes does. However, this fact sometimes gets twisted around when people are started on insulin therapy and given insufficient diabetes education and counseling. Because the eyes are sensitive to changes in blood glucose levels, it's common that when people are first diagnosed with diabetes, their vision is blurry. When they start on insulin therapy, their vision may actually worsen for a few weeks while their eyes adjust to the changes in their blood glucose level. But it's a temporary condition and, after their bodies adjust, vision improves.

Unless people are advised to expect this temporary change, some become scared and may even stop their diabetes treatment, assuming incorrectly that the insulin is causing eye problems. Through education, though, they realize that they just need to wait long enough for their bodies to adjust and stabilize to have good diabetes control and improved vision.

There are no long-term damaging side effects to using insulin. In the past, a small number of people developed allergies to components in insulin or insulin antibodies. However, with synthetic human insulin replacing insulin from animal sources, this is uncommon nowadays. The most dangerous side effect one could experience from using insulin is low blood glucose levels.

Myth #5: Diabetes is bad only if you look or feel bad.

Fact: Diabetes is a disease that everyone needs to take seriously—just like cancer is taken seriously. Would you ever tell someone that their cancer is bad only if they look bad? Of course not. We all know that if cancer isn't caught, it can spread silently throughout the body, causing problems. Likewise, diabetes isn't visible on the outside of someone's body, but inside the body it's there, and if it's not treated, it can cause problems.

Because people with diabetes look "normal," you can't tell who has it from just looking at someone. You could be sitting next to someone with diabetes and wouldn't even know it unless he or she told you. However, because the condition is a part of them, they always have it. They can't run away from it or forget about it for a day—it's with them wherever they go, to work, to school, on vacation, and on weekends. With good diabetes control, people with diabetes can otherwise be healthy and lead successful, fulfilling lives. They can look and feel great—that's the goal of diabetes treatment! But if they or you wait for them to look or feel "bad" before taking their diabetes seriously, you may regret that you've waited too long.

Myth #6: Everyone with diabetes gets complications and will go blind, lose a leg, and die. I saw it happen to someone.

Fact: This is a myth that is based on a little bit of truth, but doesn't explain all the facts. The first bit of truth is the fact that all people with diabetes will die. However, that's also true for all humans. We can't live forever.

Another truth is that people with diabetes can develop health complications such as eye, heart, kidney, and nerve problems. Diabetes is the leading cause of new cases of blindness and end-stage kidney disease. An estimated 60 to 70 percent of people with diabetes develop nerve damage, which can lead, in severe cases, to foot and leg amputations.

However, while these numbers are staggering, they represent the old age of diabetes. Not everyone is losing his or her sight or feet. As you read this, people with diabetes are rewriting their diabetes future and reducing their risk for complications. How, you may ask?

The fact is this: People with diabetes can delay or prevent complications from ever happening by keeping good blood glucose level control. With all the new medications, meters, and research to help them, they can have a different future from the one people with diabetes had just a few years ago.

Results from the Diabetes Control and Complications Trial (DCCT), published in 1993, showed that people with type 1 diabetes could lower their risk for eye, kidney, nerve, and heart disease by up to 76 percent with good long-term diabetes control. Results from the United Kingdom Prospective Diabetes Study (UKPDS) proved that people with type 2 diabetes can reduce their risk for complications, too. The UKPDS showed that those who maintain good blood glucose levels and blood pressure control can reduce their risk for stroke by 44 percent, their risk for heart failure by 56 percent, and their risk for blindness and kidney disease by 25 percent. Those with diabetes and high blood pressure found that controlling their blood pressure further reduces their risk of complications. That's exciting news!

> **Did you know** . . . *the DCCT study proved that good diabetes control could reduce the risk of complications for people with type 1 diabetes. The facts are:*
>
> *Eye disease—76% reduction*
> *Kidney disease—50% reduction*
> *Nerve disease—60% reduction*
> *Heart disease—35% reduction*

Myth #7: People with diabetes can always tell if their glucose level is high based on how they feel.

Fact: While people with diabetes may feel symptoms of low and high blood glucose levels, assessing their blood glucose level by feelings alone is neither reliable nor accurate. The only reliable way to know where someone's blood glucose level is at is to test it on a blood glucose meter. This is because sometimes a person with diabetes may feel symptoms that they think are due to diabetes for reasons totally unrelated to their disease! The only way they will know if diabetes is the cause is to test their blood glucose level. The other reason they should not trust their feelings alone is that over time, some may lose their ability to sense highs and lows. If this happens, they may develop a false confidence that their diabetes is okay when actually it's not.

Q. I've heard people say that folk remedies and herbs like aloe and garlic can cure diabetes. Do any of these really work?

A. While herbs and cultural (folk) healing methods have been practiced for centuries around the world, treatment methods called "natural," and "alternative" have not been well researched for how effective they are in promoting health, preventing disease, and improving the quality of someone's life. To date, there is no known cure for diabetes. If there were, it would make headline news and there would be no need for this book.

Until a cure is found, researchers have started to study the effects of different dietary supplements and herbs like aloe, garlic, chromium, and cactus to understand how they could be used in health promotion. However, the verdict is still out as to whether they could someday be used as a treatment for diabetes. Until they are proven to be effective and safe, and cause no harmful interactions with other medications people could use, it is best that people with diabetes discuss the use of all dietary supplements with their health care provider before considering use of them.

Q. Years ago, it seemed rare to meet someone with diabetes. But now, it seems like more and more people that I know are getting diabetes. Is something going on?

A. Diabetes is on the rise in the United States. At first, health experts thought it was due to people living longer. But now it appears to be related more to living a Western lifestyle—what people eat and how active they are.

In 1998, health experts reported that the number of people diagnosed with type 2 diabetes has increased by 9 percent every year since 1987. Between 1980 and 1994 alone, 2.2 million people were diagnosed with diabetes—an increase of 39 percent! Currently, an estimated 16 million people in the United States have diabetes. That means 6 out of every 100 people in our country have diabetes. In some ethnic groups (e.g., Native Americans, Hispanics, and African Americans), the rate is even higher.

The incidence of diabetes is also higher in older adults. Once someone reaches the age group of 65 to 74, diabetes is seen in almost one out of five people. Trends predict that soon 90 percent of those with diabetes will be over age forty-five, as roughly half of all new cases of diabetes occur in people who are over age fifty-five.

Diabetes is not just a problem in the United States. Type 2 diabetes is on the rise around the world. The World Health Organization (WHO) and the Centers for Disease Control and Prevention (CDC) are predicting that diabetes will be diagnosed in epidemic numbers in the new millennium. By the year 2025, they predict, the number of adults worldwide with diabetes will increase 122 percent, from 135 million in 1995 to 300 million. Developing countries will be affected in high numbers as they adopt Western lifestyles with eating and activity habits. By the year 2025, it's forecast that the countries most affected by diabetes will be India, China, the United States, Pakistan, Indonesia, the Russian Federation, Mexico, Brazil, Egypt, and Japan, in that order.

Besides considering the influence of the Western lifestyle, to understand the rise in diabetes, we need to look back in time to consider what else has transpired. Prior to the discovery of insulin, there were no successful long-term treatment options. If you had diabetes, it was considered a death sentence. Most lived shortened lives and had a suboptimal quality of life. This changed in 1922 with the discovery of insulin. Finally there was a treatment that worked. While it wasn't perfect, it worked to keep people alive. Couple this discovery with the advances our culture has made in technology and health care, and it has resulted in people with diabetes living longer and more productive lives than ever possible before. Thus, people are living longer with diabetes and long enough to possibly get it.

Did you know . . . over 2,200 new people are diagnosed with diabetes each day in the United States, and the rate is increasing!

Q. What are the different complications that people can get from diabetes?

A. People with diabetes are at risk for developing heart, eye, kidney, and nerve problems. While this should not be interpreted to mean that everyone with diabetes will get these complications, it means that they have a greater chance than the general population to get it. If their diabetes is poorly controlled, their risk is higher yet. Here are some of the complications that may develop.

Heart Disease

Heart disease is currently the leading cause of death among people with diabetes. Having diabetes is a risk factor for heart disease and stroke. People with diabetes are two to four times more likely to have heart disease or suffer a stroke than people without diabetes.

High Blood Pressure

It's estimated that between 60 and 65 percent of people with diabetes suffer from high blood pressure. Poorly controlled blood pressure, in turn, increases their risk for heart failure, stroke, and kidney and eye disease.

Kidney Disease

Diabetes can cause the blood vessels in the kidney to thicken, which can result in kidney damage, called *nephropathy*. If the kidneys are unable to filter the blood of the body's waste products, the waste can start to build up in the bloodstream, causing end-stage kidney disease. Left untreated, this could lead to needing dialysis or a kidney transplant.

Eye Disease

Poorly controlled diabetes can cause permanent eye damage called *retinopathy*. Retinopathy occurs when years of high blood glucose levels cause the blood vessels in the eye to leak. If not caught and treated, this can cause permanent vision loss. Currently, diabetes is the leading cause of new cases of blindness in people age 20 to 74, affecting 12,000 to 24,000 people each year.

Dental Disease

Poor diabetes control can affect the health of the mouth and teeth. It contributes to gum disease by affecting the body's ability to fight bacteria. It can also contribute to dry mouth, which is due to a decrease in saliva flow. This, in turn, can affect how well one chews or swallows food, cause a bad taste or mouth odor, and increase the risk for dental caries (cavities).

Nerve Problems

Diabetes can cause nerve damage, called *neuropathy*, and can affect different parts of the body, depending upon which area of the nervous system is affected. Peripheral neuropathy affects the nerves that reach from the spine to the outer areas of the body, like the feet and hands. This is the most common type of diabetic neuropathy affecting how the body senses things (see the lists below). For example, when bit by a mosquito, sensory nerves send signals to the brain that sense pain. When these nerves are damaged (neuropathy), legs and hands may feel numb, tingle, burn, or lose all sensation. When this happens, people may not feel pain anymore or even recognize if they injure their feet. If the injury doesn't heal, it can lead to ulcerated sores and infection. This is what commonly contributes to foot problems that end up requiring leg amputations. Each year over 56,000 amputations are performed on people with diabetes.

Did you know . . . health experts estimate that impotence affects 50 to 60 percent of men with diabetes who are over age fifty.

When neuropathy affects the autonomic system (the nerves that control basic body functions such as the heart, bladder, and intestinal systems), it can sometimes affect the stomach and intestines, causing bowel irregularity, nausea, and vomiting. Other times, it can affect the urinary tract or sexual organs, causing impotence, vaginal dryness, or urination problems. It's estimated that 60 to 70 percent of people with diabetes will develop some form of nerve damage, whether mild or severe, during their lifetime.

Common Signs of Peripheral Neuropathy

- tingling
- burning sensations
- loss of feeling in hands or feet
- loss of ability to sense hot or cold temperatures
- poor balance
- foot deformities
- poor healing, open sores on the feet

Common Signs of Autonomic Neuropathy

- frequent urinary tract infections
- difficulty urinating or incontinence
- impotence
- decreased vaginal fluids
- diarrhea and constipation
- early satiety while eating
- delayed stomach emptying
- dry hands and feet
- upper body sweating

Q. What tests do doctors commonly order when someone has diabetes?

A. When someone has diabetes, doctors may do a variety of tests to monitor how their blood glucose control has been and whether the diabetes has started to cause any complications. Here are a few common tests that a doctor may order:

***Glycosylated Hemoglobin Test** (also known as glycated hemoglobin, hemoglobin A1, hemoglobin A1c, or HbA1c)*
This test is often done three to four times a year and helps reflect how well someone's blood glucose control has been over the past two to three months. The test consists of taking a small blood sample and measuring it in a lab to find out much glucose is attached to the blood's hemoglobin (the part of a red blood cell that carries oxygen). The higher the level of glucose in the blood, the more glucose that attaches to the hemoglobin. A normal HbA1c level ranges 4 to 6 percent. Diabetes control is considered good when the HbA1c level is at or below 7 percent. To determine what someone's average blood glucose level was from the HbA1c result, see the table on page 42.

***Glycosylated Albumin** (fructosamine)*
This test may be done after someone has changed their diabetes treatment program to assess how well it's working. It measures the average blood glucose level over a two-to-three-week period.

Lipid Panel
This fasting blood test helps assess one's risk for heart disease. It measures one's total cholesterol, HDL cholesterol, LDL cholesterol, and triglyceride level.

WHAT DOES THE HbA1c NUMBER MEAN?		
HbA1c Level (%)	Average Blood Glucose Level (mg/dl) Over Past 2–3 Months*	Diabetes Control
6	120	Ideal
7	150	Good
8	180	Fair
9	210	Poor
10	240	Poor
11	270	Poor
12	300	Poor
13	330	Poor

Note: Results may vary from one testing lab to another and whether one has erratic (many low and high) glucose levels.

Adapted with Permission from *Diabetes Self-Management.* ©1998, R.A. Rapaport Publishing, Inc. For sample copy call 800/234-0923.

Urine Analysis

The doctor may require a urine specimen to assess how well the kidneys are functioning. They commonly check to see if there is any protein, creatinine, or microalbumin that may have spilled into the urine, which is a marker of how well the kidneys are working.

Other Tests

Eye Dilation: Because the eye is sensitive to high blood glucose levels in the body, doctors routinely check the eye's retina for any eye disease that may develop. By catching problems early, prompt eye treatment can preserve eyesight.

Blood Pressure: Uncontrolled high blood pressure can increase one's risk for heart disease and stroke. In some people, it can reflect kidney disease. Because of this, health care providers regularly monitor blood pressure levels.

Foot Inspection: Over time, some people with diabetes develop a loss of sensation in their feet. They may not notice when shoes fit poorly or if they step on something that causes a sore. When diabetes control is poor, foot sores are slow to heal.

Because of this, doctors will inspect the feet of people with diabetes to promote good foot health and catch foot problems before they get out of control.

Q. What are the AGEs that researchers have started to test for?

A. Research is looking for common traits among people who develop diabetes complications. So far, it looks as if *advanced glycation end products* (AGEs) may be one such trait. Here's how.

When people have poor diabetes control, their high glucose levels cause wear and tear on the body tissues and protein. When protein in the body is exposed to high levels of glucose over long periods of time, it becomes altered, which produces AGEs. These compounds can affect collagen, which can cause cell membranes to become stiff and leak. In turn, this is thought to contribute to the development of diabetes complications.

Scientists are looking for ways to test for AGEs and stop them from forming.

Did you know . . . *for every percentage point reduction in their glycosylated hemoglobin (HbA1c) level, people can reduce their risk for eye, kidney, and nerve damage by 35 percent.*

Q. My wife was just diagnosed with gestational diabetes. Does this mean she will have diabetes for the rest of her life?

A. Gestational diabetes is a temporary form of diabetes that is diagnosed during pregnancy. After the birth of the baby, nine out of ten women find that their blood glucose level returns to normal—their diabetes disappears. However, a few women will continue to have trouble with glucose. They will go on to have either impaired glucose tolerance or type 2 diabetes.

For the women who have their blood glucose level return to normal, they need to know that they are at risk for developing diabetes in the future. With future pregnancies, they may develop gestational diabetes again. If they are overweight, they are at high risk for developing a glucose impairment or type 2 diabetes later in life.

Q. My mom and one uncle have type 2 diabetes. How can I tell if I'm at risk for getting it, too?

A. To determine your risk for developing type 2 diabetes, complete the quiz below. The more questions you answer yes to, the higher your risk.

Self-Assessment Quiz

Directions: Check the response, either "yes" or "no," that best answers the following questions.

	Yes	No
1. Are you over 45 years old?	☐	☐
2. Do you have a biological parent, sibling, or close relative who has diabetes?	☐	☐
3. Are you currently overweight?	☐	☐
4. Do you have high blood pressure?	☐	☐
5. Are you generally inactive? (accumulate less than 30 minutes of physical activity every day)	☐	☐
6. Are you of Native American, Asian, Hispanic, African American, or Pacific Islander ethnic background?	☐	☐
7. Have you ever had gestational diabetes or given birth to a baby weighing over nine pounds?	☐	☐

Interpreting Your Results: If you answered "yes" to at least two of the questions above, start now to make changes in your eating habits and activity level to reduce your risk. See your doctor to have your blood glucose level checked on a regular basis.

Q. What are the odds that I could get diabetes if my mother has it?

A. If you had no risk factors marked on the quiz, your risk for getting diabetes is small. How small, you may wonder? Generally, only three or four (0.3–0.4%) people out of every thousand in our country develop some form of diabetes. However, if diabetes runs in your family, your risk level goes up. If you have a brother or sister with type 1 diabetes, your risk rises to 5 to 6 percent. If you have a parent with type 1 diabetes, your risk is 2 to 6 percent. Your risk for developing type 2 diabetes if one of your parents or siblings has diabetes is 40 percent. If you had gestational diabetes, your risk for type 2 diabetes or a glucose impairment jumps to 50 percent!

As you consider your risk level for getting diabetes, remember that these are your odds based upon survey and research data. Heredity is only one factor that can contribute to your chance of getting diabetes. Don't forget to factor in the role you contribute and can put either in your favor or against you. If you are overweight, sedentary, and live a lifestyle that is not healthy, your risk for developing diabetes can go up. To decrease your risk for diabetes, start taking steps today to change the factors you can control. When you eat healthy and exercise regularly, consider it diabetes insurance you're doing for yourself.

Q. Where can I go if I want to learn more about diabetes?

A. To learn more about diabetes, how it's treated, and the complications people can develop from it, see the suggested additional reading list at the back of the book.

CHAPTER 2

Managing Low Blood Glucose

WHAT IF HE HAS A DIABETES INSULIN REACTION WHILE I'M WITH HIM?
WHAT SHOULD I DO? HOW CAN I HELP?

Have you ever worried about what you would do if someone with diabetes had an insulin reaction while you were with him or her? If you have, you're not alone. It's natural for friends and family to worry about this, especially if they've never experienced it. Sometimes the worry and anticipation imagining what could happen are worse than reality when you don't know what to expect.

The good news is, with a little education and pre-planning, you can learn what to expect and how to calm your fears. In this chapter, you will learn what hypoglycemia is, what causes it, and how to treat it when it happens. You will also learn how it can be prevented.

Let's start with the basics.

Q. What is hypoglycemia?

A. Hypoglycemia literally means "low blood glucose." The term is used to describe a condition where someone's blood glucose level is below normal. Hypoglycemia, more commonly called a reaction or insulin reaction, a low sugar level, or insulin shock, is a negative side effect of having diabetes.

Hypoglycemia is most likely to affect those people who use insulin to treat their diabetes. While those using diabetes pills can have occasional lows, it is unlikely if they follow their prescribed meal plan and take their diabetes medication on schedule. Lows are uncommon in those who are able to manage their diabetes solely through lifestyle efforts—diet, exercise, and maintaining a desirable weight.

Q. What causes hypoglycemia?

A. Hypoglycemia is caused by having too much insulin and too little glucose in the bloodstream at the same time. Low blood glucose levels occur most often around mealtimes (right before or during a meal) and during or after strenuous exercise. This can often be attributed to changes in a person's habits or usual schedule. For example, lows can happen as a result of:

- Delaying or skipping a meal or snack.
- Eating less food than usual (especially carbohydrates).
- Taking too much insulin or diabetes pills.
- Exercising longer or harder than usual.
- Drinking alcohol on an empty stomach.

Q. What happens when someone's blood glucose level is low? What symptoms do they feel?

A. When blood glucose levels drop below 70 mg/dl—the lowest level considered normal—a person may start feeling a range of mild physical, mental, and/or emotional symptoms (see the table on page 49.) At first the symptoms (warning signs) are mostly noticeable just to the person having them. Because each person with diabetes is different, what one person feels when low can vary slightly from what somebody else feels. It's interesting that from time to time, the symptoms felt can even vary within the same person, depending upon the situation.

When glucose levels drop below 60 mg/dl, a person will start to experience symptoms where they may sense something is wrong with their body. They may start to feel sweaty, shaky, nervous, or like their lips are tingling. As their glucose level continues to drop, these symptoms become noticeable to people around them as their muscle coordination and mood become affected. A person with low glucose may start acting as if he or she is drunk—walking with a staggered gait, acting giddy, and having slower reflexes. Some may even look confused or like they're in a trance, staring into space, unable to focus on anything, or unable to hold a meaningful conversation. Were their blood glucose level to continue dropping, they could pass out and eventually even die. However, when hypoglycemia is treated promptly, the good news is that the symptoms will go away as the blood glucose level returns to normal.

How can I help? Ask the person you know with diabetes to describe how he feels when he has low blood glucose. By knowing what warning signs you may spot him having, you'll be able to help him catch and maybe prevent a low from happening!

Q. If someone's glucose level drops below 30 mg/dl, is it true that it could cause brain damage? Just how dangerous is hypoglycemia?

A. When treating hypoglycemia, the biggest concern people with diabetes face is not so much how low they go (what number they get down to), but rather how long the low lasts before it's treated. While all hypoglycemia episodes have the potential to become dangerous, mild episodes are often considered by people with diabetes to be more of a nuisance and an unpleasant side effect of having diabetes that they accept. Usually, they are able to treat mild lows themselves (without asking for help) and continue their normal activities. (See page 50 for treatment tips.)

Hypoglycemia becomes more serious when blood glucose levels drop to the point where the brain starts to run low on glucose. When this happens, it starts to affect physical coordination and the ability to think clearly. If they are operating equipment

Signs and Symptoms of Low Blood Glucose

Overall Hypogly-cemia Severity	Glucose Level	Symptoms They May Feel	Signs You May See
Mild	Below 60 mg/dl	Anxious	Anxiety
		Dizzy/lightheaded/shaky	Wobbly/poor balance
		Fast pulse	
		Hungry	
		Nauseous	
		Nervous	Nervous habits
		Sweaty	Perspiration; cold, clammy skin
		Tingling lips/mouth	
Moderate	Below 40 mg/dl	Blurred vision	Difficulty reading or seeing
		Confusion	Inability to talk logically; unable to solve problems
		Drowsy	Sleepy
		Headaches	Rubbing their temples
		Lack of coordination; delayed reflexes	Poor physical coordination; slurred speech; staggered gait; poor hand–eye coordination
		Mood changes—irritability, anger, sadness, impatience, giddiness	Inappropriate or unexpected mood change; unusual stubbornness, anger, silliness, crying, pessimistic attitude, impatience
		Nightmares	Tossing or turning in their sleep; crying out in their sleep
		Stupor	Trancelike look (spacy); glassy-eyed look
Severe	Below 20 mg/dl	Convulsions	Seizures
		Delirium	Irrational behavior, delirious, wandering, unable to talk clearly
		Faint (pass out)	Unconsciousness

or driving an automobile when this happens, the situation becomes potentially dangerous because their reflexes may be slower, which puts them at risk for possibly injuring themselves and/or hurting others. Were they to reach a point where they couldn't self-treat a low, the situation could turn very dangerous. Unless they receive help promptly, their glucose level could continue to drop. If the low glucose level results in them passing out for a long period of time (minutes versus hours), the brain cells could become permanently damaged. They could even experience convulsions and die from a low left untreated.

Q. How is hypoglycemia treated? How can I help?

A. Yes, you can help someone treat hypoglycemia. Treating low blood glucose isn't scary or hard to do. How you can help will depend upon how alert the person having the low is. If he or she is alert, you can help find food or beverages that contain carbohydrates (sugar) they can eat. However, if they are unable to treat themselves or are unconscious, they will need your help to receive emergency medical care that may consist of helping them eat food, giving them a glucagon injection (see page 55), or calling 911 for emergency care.

Helping treat lows is easy if you follow these three rules:

Rule #1: If in doubt, test it out!
If someone with diabetes wonders if her glucose level could be low because she feels symptoms (or you're spotting warning signs—see page 49), encourage her to test her blood to find out. The first rule of treating lows is, *"If in doubt, test it out."* Testing should never be considered a waste of time or effort. Through testing, you'll both know in less than a minute (the time it takes for a blood glucose meter to analyze a blood sample) whether her level is low, normal, or high.

If you spot her having warning signs of a low and aren't sure how to approach her about testing, don't be shy. It's better to speak up and show your concern than keep silent and run the risk that she has a low that could have been prevented or caught early. Remember, you're asking her to test because you care about her and her health.

An easy way to approach her and start a conversation about her health is to show your concern and ask how she feels. Let her know you noticed she isn't looking her usual self and describe what you observed. If she agrees that she's not feeling her best, quietly ask whether she could have a low glucose level. If she agrees she could, encourage her to test her blood to see where she's at, if she hasn't done so already.

After she tests, you'll both feel more confident because you've taken action to check on her health. If her glucose level turns out to be normal, you'll both know that diabetes isn't the cause of the symptoms. Together you can then look for other reasons that explain how she's feeling. For example, if she is feeling shaky and sweaty before giving a speech in front of a large group, then her symptoms are not due to diabetes but probably to her body's normal response to stress. If, however, her glucose level turns out to be low, feel good that you've helped her catch a low and shown her that you care.

Rule #2: Treat lows using the "15/15 Rule."

The goal of treating hypoglycemia is to return the blood glucose level to normal as soon as possible. However, in the rush to treat a low, sometimes people panic and follow the old cliché "If a little is good, more is better." While this concept may work with kneading bread or buffing a car so it's shiny, it doesn't work well for treating hypoglycemia, as it leads to overtreatment.

Overtreating a low blood glucose level can send it skyrocketing, causing a rebound high blood glucose level that will fall later on. A rebound creates a rollercoaster effect, where the glucose level drops low and then swings high and back down again. This effect can prolong the time it takes for the person to totally recover from a hypoglycemia episode. To prevent overtreating lows, follow the "15/15 rule" to play it safe.

15/15 Rule

1. *Eat 15 grams* of carbohydrate (see the list on page 53)—this amount has the potential to raise blood glucose levels 45 points.

2. *Wait 15 minutes* for the treatment to take effect—usually they will start to feel better within a few minutes.

3. *Recheck* the blood glucose level (if you're able to) to make sure it has returned to her target range.

4. *Repeat* steps 1 through 3 if she is still having symptoms or her glucose level is still below 70 mg/dl. Once her level returns to normal, have her start eating her meal as soon as possible if the low happened right before a meal. If the low occurred between meals, encourage her to eat a small snack to tide her over until her next meal so her glucose level doesn't go low again.

The most challenging part of treating lows is having the patience to wait for the carbohydrate to work. It will be hard for both you and the person with diabetes to wait, because you want her to feel better as soon as possible. And until that happens, each minute will seem to last forever. But remember, it's important to be patient and give the treatment time to work. Once she eats 15 grams of carbohydrate, it can take the body from five to fifteen minutes to digest the food and turn it into glucose. If you encourage her to eat until her symptoms go away, you'll find that she can eat a lot of food in fifteen minutes. Overeating leads to overtreating and rebound high blood glucose levels later on, and can promote unwanted weight gain.

As a rule of thumb, the 15-gram carbohydrate treatment amount works well for most people and is a simple number to remember. However, just as there are often two roads that can lead to the same place, there are sometimes variations on how much carbohydrate people need to effectively treat a low. Those on an intensive insulin therapy program aiming for tight control and who frequently test their blood glucose level may be advised by their doctor to treat their lows with less carbohydrate during the day and more during the night. This is because their treatment amount is tailored to their unique diabetes needs. If, however, you are unsure how much carbohydrate the person you know with diabetes uses to treat lows, you can't go wrong by playing it safe and offering 15 grams.

When looking for food choices that contain carbohydrate to use as treatment, use the carbohydrate information provided on food labels in the *Nutrition Facts* area. There are two things to consider when reading food label information. First, choose food items that are high in carbohydrate and low in protein and fat that are convenient to find and keep on hand. Second, consider items made from glucose or that have a high glycemic index. For example, flavored glucose tablets and gels in a tube can be purchased inexpensively in drugstores and used as a convenient treatment choice. Because they are made from glucose, the body is able to digest them a little faster than other forms of sugar, like those found in fruit and table sugar. While we're only talking about a difference in seconds or a few minutes, many with diabetes find using glucose tablets a nice option when they're away from home or traveling and don't want to carry perishable food with them to be used as potential treatment choices.

Foods with Roughly 15* Grams of Carbohydrate

- 3–4 glucose tablets (varies per brand)
- 4 sugar cubes or sugar packets
- 1 tablespoon honey, corn syrup, jelly, or frosting
- ½ cup regular cola or soft drink
- 3 graham cracker squares
- 1 slice of bread
- ½ cup orange juice
- ¾ cup dry, ready-to-eat breakfast cereal (e.g., Rice Krispies, Chex, Cheerios)

*Note: Because carbohydrate contents can vary among food products, these amounts are rough averages of different products. For more accurate measures, refer to the Nutrition Facts section of a product's food label to determine the exact carbohydrate amount of a serving. If you need to treat with partial servings, aim for a total carbohydrate amount that is between 10 and 15 grams to prevent overtreating. For people using acarbose (an anti-diabetes pill), glucose tablets and gels work best.

*Rule #3: If They Can't Swallow or Have Passed Out,
Give Them Glucagon or Call 911.*

If someone's glucose level drops so low that he is no longer able to treat himself because he is confused, sleepy, uncooperative, or has passed out, you'll need to act quickly to help him out. Follow these emergency guidelines:

- Check to see if he is conscious. If he is conscious, but confused or in a trancelike state, have him sit in a safe location where he cannot fall or hurt himself.

- Next, determine if he is able to swallow. If he can, try placing some glucose gel, honey, jelly, sugar, or syrup inside his cheek. If he is unable to swallow, do not place food or liquids in his mouth.

- If he is awake but uncooperative or unable to swallow, give him an injection of glucagon if a glucagon kit is available (see page 55). If glucagon is not available or he fails to respond to glucagon, call for emergency medical help (dial 911 in most cities).

- If he is unconscious, place him on his side in a recovery position by rolling him over onto his side (turn his head, shoulders, and torso in unison to prevent twisting). Placing him in this position ensures that his airway stays open and he won't suffocate by having his tongue fall back and block his windpipe. If glucagon is available, give him an injection immediately. If glucagon isn't available or he fails to respond to it, call for emergency medical help (dial 911 in most cities).

What Not to Do

- Don't wait to see if he'll get better on his own before taking action—this will only delay getting him the help he might need.

- Don't treat lows by giving insulin or diabetes medication—this will result in his glucose level going lower.

■ Don't force food or liquids down his throat if he is not awake—this can lead to choking and aspiration pneumonia.

Did you know . . . sometimes when people with diabetes feel a low coming on, they delay treatment until they're finished with a project or everyone is present to start eating a meal together. Thinking they can wait just a little while longer, they run the risk of experiencing a more severe reaction. Unfortunately, waiting doesn't work. Treating a low should be considered a number one priority by all—promote safety first.

Q. What is glucagon?

A. Glucagon is a hormone made by the pancreas that works opposite to insulin. When blood glucose levels are low, the pancreas senses this. In response, it makes and releases glucagon into the bloodstream to signal the body to release glucose into the bloodstream from cells and tissues, thus raising the glucose level.

Because researchers have figured out a way to make glucagon, it can be purchased in small emergency kits that friends and family members can use to help treat low blood glucose levels that result in someone not being alert enough to swallow or being unconscious. Consisting of a small bottle of glucagon powder and a syringe prefilled with liquid, glucagon kits are easy to use. You can quickly activate the powder by adding the liquid in the syringe to the bottle and mixing. Next, you simply draw up the glucagon solution back into the syringe and inject it into the person with low blood glucose.

Glucagon can be injected almost anywhere in the body. The results are quick. In an adult, an injection usually takes effect within five to twenty minutes and should raise someone's glucose level 20–30 mg/dl to a level where he becomes conscious again. However, because the effects are short-lasting, once he is alert enough to eat, you'll need to encourage him to eat a small snack to ensure that his glucose level stays up.

If this is the first you've heard about glucagon, it's important to take a few minutes to learn how to use a glucagon kit and give an injection if you have a friend or family member who uses insulin to treat his diabetes. Consider the time you spend learning to use the kit an investment or emergency insurance plan for yourself and him so you feel prepared to use the kit if an emergency arises. Remember, when severe hypoglycemia occurs, you won't be able to ask the person with diabetes how to use the kit. He won't be able to show you. Thus, learning how to use the kit will help you gain confidence that you can help someone treat hypoglycemia.

Be prepared . . . if someone you know uses insulin, ask if he has a glucagon kit. If he doesn't have one, encourage him to get one. Store the kit in a location that is easily accessible and remember to let everyone around know where the kit is stored. Then, once a year, check the kit's expiration date and replace it when it is old.

If you need help learning how to use glucagon and syringes, talk with a certified diabetes educator or your friend's diabetes health care provider. Most educators have access to sample glucagon kits and syringes you can practice with. Through practicing, you'll feel confident in your skills and someday may end up saving your friend or relative an expensive trip to a hospital emergency room.

Q. What should I do if my wife thinks she's low, but she doesn't have a meter around to test and I can't remember the 15/15 rule?

A. In the midst of treating a possible low, if she doesn't have a meter and you can't remember all the rules for treating hypoglycemia, it's wise to have a backup plan. There are two golden rules that make up a backup plan for the three treatment rules described above. If you remember these rules, in times of doubt you'll always be prepared.

Golden Rule #1: If someone has symptoms but can't test, treat all potential lows

There may be times when the person you know feels low but doesn't have a meter nearby to check his glucose level. If this happens, he should follow the first golden rule of hypoglycemia, which is to treat all potential lows. Error on the side of safety and treat rather than risk not treating a possible low.

Golden Rule #2: If in doubt about what to give, treat with something sweet (sugar)

If you're helping someone treat a low but you're unsure what food to offer, pick food or liquid that is sweet or high in sugar. The body will make glucose quickest from foods high in carbohydrate such as hard candy, sweetened beverages, bread, fruit, or crackers. Avoid giving high-fat or -protein foods (e.g., meat, cheese, nuts, ice cream, or chocolate candy bars), as they take longer to break down into glucose in the body and are less effective.

How can I help? Learn the rules for treating lows!

Rule #1: *If in doubt, test it out!*
  Golden Rule #1: *If they have symptoms but can't test, treat all potential lows.*
Rule #2: *Treat lows using the 15/15 rule.*
  Golden Rule #2: *If in doubt what to give, treat with something sweet (sugar).*
Rule #3: *If they can't swallow or have passed out, give them glucagon or call 911.*

Q. My wife doesn't think she needs to test her blood glucose level because she says she can always sense when it's low. However, I don't think she can, because I often notice she's low before she does. Is her diabetes getting worse if she can't sense lows well anymore?

A. While it's true that people with diabetes can learn to sense when their blood glucose level is really high or low, total reliance on feelings alone is not safe. It can cause one to develop a false sense of security about their diabetes.

When people rely on feelings alone, they may believe that as long as they don't feel low, they aren't low. However, no one can predict with complete accuracy where their blood glucose level is at. It's impossible. It's like predicting how much air is in a car tire. You may sense (by sight or feel) that a tire on your car is getting flat or has plenty of air in it, but you need to use a tire gauge to find out what the air level really is. As you drive, you need to periodically recheck the air level as a safety check to ensure that the tires are properly inflated. Similarly, the best way to know exactly where someone's blood glucose level is at is to use a reliable testing tool (i.e., a blood glucose meter). Symptoms of low blood glucose only alert someone that their glucose level may be abnormal—symptoms don't quantify the level where someone is at.

Another reason why people shouldn't rely on feelings alone to know where their blood glucose level is, is that over time people can lose the ability to sense the early warning signs of hypoglycemia. When this happens, it's called *hypoglycemic unawareness*.

Because people with hypoglycemic unawareness are no longer able to sense lows like they used to, it's common for other people to start noticing they are low before they do. They could even pass out from a low without sensing anything is going to happen. Because of this, they can't rely on their senses. Instead, they need to rely on regular blood glucose testing and on friends and family members to spot warning signs that they have hypoglycemia.

If your wife develops hypoglycemic unawareness, does it mean her diabetes is worse? No. It just looks that way because instead of catching lows when they're mild (not noticeable to others), she is catching them at levels lower than she did before, where the symptoms and warning signs are more noticeable. Consequently, when she identifies her blood glucose level as low, it's doubly important that she treats promptly. Otherwise, she may reach a level where she passes out if she and those around her fail to notice that she is low. One moment she could be talking to you and the next minute—poof—she's lying on the ground unconscious. For safety's sake, it's important that people with hypoglycemic unawareness:

How can I help? Encourage the person with diabetes you care about to not rely on feelings alone to know where their glucose level is. Encourage testing on a regular basis.

- test blood glucose levels more often and in a consistent manner

- ask friends and family members to watch for signs of hypoglycemia

- maintain a slightly higher target blood glucose range to reduce their risk of serious lows (if they haven't done this, they should talk with their health care provider about how to do this)

- be extra careful to not delay or skip meals and snacks

Q. My husband is usually a gentle, quiet person, but when his blood glucose level is low he gets ornery and stubborn. Is it normal for someone's personality to change during a reaction? If so, why does this happen?

A. Yes. When blood glucose levels are low, it's common for someone to experience personality or mood changes. Remember, the body runs on glucose for energy—this includes the brain. When the brain cells run low on glucose, it affects their ability to work correctly. This results in a person being unable to think clearly. Consequently when someone is hypoglycemic, you may notice them acting differently or changing moods. Suddenly—or so it can seem—a person who is usually polite, gentle, and considerate could become angry or uncooperative. They may become more stubborn than usual or lose their patience easily.

Because the changes in their physical and emotional behavior are a result of their brain not getting enough glucose, the changes are reversible once their hypoglycemia is treated. As their glucose level returns to normal, usually so does their mood.

When your husband is in the midst of treating a low blood glucose level, you need to remember that he may not be thinking clearly because of the low. This can cause him to behave in ways he usually wouldn't and even

> *Did you know . . . those who rely on their feelings alone to know whether their diabetes is under control usually don't have the best control.*

argue with you. Try not to take what is said personally or to heart. While it may seem hurtful or abrupt, it's usually not intentional.

Sometime when your husband is feeling well, share with him your concern about how he acts when he has a low. Explain how you dislike arguing with him when he's low. Find out if he's aware of his mood changes and how it affects you. If he isn't aware of this, you'll need to explain what happens so he understands the frustration you feel.

While he can't promise to never be moody when he's low, you can work together to prevent and treat his lows effectively and calmly. Ask him for ideas on how you can best help him treat his lows when he is acting stubborn. Make a pact to not hold serious family discussions or make expensive financial decisions during or right after a low—agree to give him a few minutes to recover first. He's bound to appreciate your sensitivity and understanding of what he feels when he has a low. This way, you'll feel more relaxed and able to focus on the important conversations you want to have with each other and avoid unnecessary arguments.

Q. I've noticed that my fiancé becomes closed-minded when he's having an insulin reaction. If I ask if he wants a treatment, he will snap at me, saying "no" when he isn't really sure what he wants. How should I handle this when it happens?

A. The next time your fiancé's glucose level is low and he isn't able to think clearly as to how he is going to treat himself, it's important that you recognize the fact that he needs help. At this point, you need to take control of the situation and get him to eat or drink something. Be gentle with him, but firmly coax him to eat. Try these tips next time:

1. *Control your emotions—stay calm and neutral.* Remember, if he says something hurtful to you, don't take it personally, as it's the low blood glucose level that's talking, not him.

2. *Assess the situation at hand.* Determine whether he is able to test his own blood glucose level or not. If he is, gently but firmly ask him to test to learn exactly where his glucose level is at. If his blood glucose meter is close at hand, help him test his level. If it isn't possible to test, go ahead and start treating the low. If time is of the essence, start treating the low and test afterward.

3. *When someone is unable to treat himself, don't waste time asking him what food he wants to eat for his treatment; make the decision for him.* If you ask him to make decisions during a low, he may say "no" when you'd expect him to say "yes." This is because saying "no" is often the easiest answer to give when feeling confused or unable to focus on a conversation. So bring him food or liquid high in carbohydrate. Encourage him to consume it to treat his low. If he says "no" and doesn't want to eat what you bring, ask him why not. If he's unable to explain clearly why he doesn't want to eat the food, it's the low talking to you—you'll need to encourage him to eat the food you've brought him. However, if he can clearly tell you why he doesn't want the food you brought and is able to suggest an acceptable alternative, rest assured that he's not so low that he isn't able to treat himself.

4. *If in doubt as to what food to give, offer a sweetened soft drink, juice, or a favorite sweet treat close at hand that he usually enjoys eating.* If he already likes a food or beverage, he'll be more apt to consume it than reject it. With experience helping to treat lows, you'll soon learn which foods you can coax him into eating most easily and can keep those on hand for use as treatments.

5. *If he's dazed or needs prompting to eat, stand to his side or in front of him and gently but firmly urge him to eat the food or drink the liquid.* Don't be afraid to be assertive. For example:

If he's ornery, try:

- *"Tell me what you think of this. Try a bite (sip)."*—Say this to coax (persuade) him to eat a favorite food or drink.

- *"I got this especially for you. Have a bite—you'll feel better soon."*—Say this if he needs encouragement to eat.

- *"I got some of your favorite juice and brought you a glass, too. Have a sip."*—Say this if you want to casually coax him to drink.

If he's dazed, try :

- *"Here, I think you need to eat this."*—Say this as you either hand him the food or help him guide the food toward his mouth.

- *"Let me help you take a sip."*—Say this if he is dazed and not sure how to drink what you bring him.

- *"That's it, chew it up—chew, chew, chew."*—Say this if he is forgetting to chew after he puts the food in his mouth.

6. Continue coaxing him to eat/sip the food until he's finished the portion. Follow the 15/15 rule to avoid overtreating the low (see page 52).

Remember, if he's unable to swallow on his own, don't force food or pour liquid down his throat, as it could lead to choking or aspiration. Aspiration is when food goes down the windpipe into the lungs instead of down the esophagus into the stomach. Aspiration can cause pneumonia (inflammation of the lungs). If he is unable to swallow or is uncooperative, give him an injection of glucagon. The glucagon should arouse him enough to make him feel better and more receptive to helping you treat his low.

Q. I always thought my wife, who has type 1 diabetes, had good blood glucose control because she never has lows. Is this correct? How often do people usually have lows?

A. That's a question with many answers. In general, it's impossible to assess how good a person's diabetes control is based solely on whether they are having lows or not. To assess diabetes control, you need to consider other factors as well; for example, what type of diabetes they have, how it's being treated, and their lifestyle. If you don't consider these facts, you won't see the full picture of how well their diabetes is under control. Remember, good control is avoiding low and high blood glucose levels.

People who do not use insulin to treat their diabetes are at lower risk for having lows; thus, they'll have fewer episodes. For those, however, who treat their diabetes with insulin and are trying to achieve tight glucose control, they may experience mild hypoglycemia as often as once or twice a week. When it happens, they can usually pinpoint the reason for the low. For them, mild lows are just a side effect of keeping their glucose level as close to normal as possible. Over time, most learn to prevent and catch the lows when they are mild by testing their blood glucose level regularly.

However, when lows happen frequently—at night while sleeping or for unknown reasons—it should be a signal that the diabetes treatment plan needs review and possible adjustment. By reviewing with their health care provider the pattern of the lows they're having, they can determine if their target goal or insulin doses need to be changed. Their doctor may modify or raise their target glucose range to help protect them from lows if they have hypoglycemic unawareness or can't sense when they're low.

How can I help? Encourage people with diabetes to strive for good blood glucose control by seeing their health care provider on a regular basis. They should review their treatment plan and make periodic adjustments to reflect changes in their lifestyles and habits.

Q. When I golf with my roommate, he often has insulin reactions while we're walking the course. However, if I'm winning, he blames his game on his diabetes and robs from me the satisfaction of knowing I beat him fair and square. Is there something he could do to prevent the reactions?

A. No one likes a sore loser, especially one who makes excuses about why he didn't win instead of congratulating the person who did. However, the fact remains that hypoglycemia is an inconvenient and potentially disruptive side effect of diabetes. When it happens, it tends to interrupt whatever people are doing—even golf games. So, when hypoglycemia occurs, it's something people have to deal with quickly. Treatment takes top priority over all other things going on—whether it's finishing a game of golf or a project.

Consequently, it's true that if your roommate has a reaction while he's exercising, he may not play his best level of golf for a few minutes. However, if he's frequently having lows while golfing, encourage him to discuss it with his health care provider. Through education and learning exercise self-management skills, there are ways he can plan ahead for golf outings and prevent lows from happening to ensure that he's always feeling his best.

People with good diabetes control tend to experience lower glucose levels with exercise. Therefore, to prevent lows during or after exercising, they need to remember to plan ahead. If they know they're going to be exercising at a certain time of the day, they may be able to reduce or adjust the amount of insulin they take to compensate. For exercise or activity that is unplanned, they may compensate for the effect of exercise by eating a small carbohydrate-rich snack. Depending on how long they exercise and how strenuous the exercise is, they may need to snack before, during, and after their workout to prevent their glucose level from falling too low. The snack may consist of fruit, crackers, a glass of milk or juice, or even a small sandwich if they are planning to exercise strenuously over a long period of time.

If someone has poor diabetes control, exercise can cause blood glucose levels to rise. How could this happen? Well, when blood glucose levels are over 240 mg/dl, it's a sign that the body could be having trouble using glucose for energy. To know for sure, it's necessary to test one's urine for ketones. If ketones are present, it means the body is low on insulin and has started to use fatty acids for energy instead of glucose. In this situation, exercise will cause the blood glucose levels to go higher as the body will release glucose for the cells to use as energy—only they aren't able to use it due to the lack of insulin. If however, ketones are not present in the urine, the body has sufficient insulin to normalize the glucose level, and exercise is safe to do.

You can help your roommate prevent hypoglycemia by encouraging him to test his glucose level before he golfs. Between rounds of golf, offer to take a quick break. This will allow him the chance to retest his glucose level and grab a snack or beverage if he needs to. For extra safety, consider carrying a package of glucose tablets or something sweet in your golf bag that you can offer as a treatment should his glucose level get low while you're out on the golf course.

Did you know . . . if someone's glucose level is over 240 mg/dl, they need to be cautious exercising because doing so could cause his level to go higher. When blood glucose levels are high, it means that the cells are not using the glucose for energy because of a problem with insulin. If he exercises, it will cause his body to make and release glucose into his bloodstream for muscles and cells to use as energy. However, this only leads to higher blood glucose levels, because the underlying insulin problem still exists.

Q. I'm getting married next month and my fiancée has type 1 diabetes. Could she have an insulin reaction while we have sex?

A. Yes. As mentioned above, physical activity and exercise have the potential to lower someone's glucose level. So if sexual activity occurs over an extended time period and/or disrupts your fiancée's usual mealtimes, she could experience a low.

If you are worried about this happening, you need to share your concern with your fiancée. Otherwise, you could end up worrying about this during your honeymoon and married life for years to come, which could detract from your enjoying intimate times together. Working together, though, you can take steps to prevent lows from happening. Here's how.

- If you're planning for sexual activities to occur at a certain time and she is on an intensive insulin therapy program, she may want to adjust her insulin dose or the size of her meal to compensate, as taught by her health care provider.

- If the sexual activities are unplanned (spontaneous), she may want to eat a quick snack before or afterward. Keep a few items next to your bed in a nightstand that are high in carbohydrate that can be used as a quick hypoglycemia treatment or exercise snack. For example, try keeping an individual juice or sweetened fruit drink box or glucose tabs. That way if she has a low after sex or even during the night, she has food readily available for her use. This also helps minimize the risk of you or her stubbing a toe or banging a shin into something (furniture or items left on the floor) when rushing to the kitchen to get food for a treatment. Accidental injuries caused by rushing are almost guaranteed to break up any romantic mood—much more so than the treatment of mild hypoglycemia.

Q. Once before an office lunch meeting, I was shocked to see an officemate, who has type 1 diabetes, rip open a packet of sugar and pour the contents into a spoon so she could eat it. I watched her eat a couple of packets right in a row! I thought people with diabetes were supposed to avoid sugar. Should I have confronted her?

A. Because people don't commonly eat spoonfuls of sugar, you observed an unusual sight. Because the person who did it had diabetes and it occurred before a meal, it's reasonable to guess that your officemate may have been self-treating a low blood glucose level. Using sugar packets to treat hypoglycemia is a method many people with diabetes use when dining out and their meal is late being served. Using sugar packets also allows people to quickly treat their low glucose level instead of having to flag a waiter to rush them food or juice to drink. Sugar packets are a convenient treatment option, as they are readily accessible (usually right on the table), easy to use, come in preportioned packages, and are effective. After eating the sugar, they can then calmly catch a waiter as he goes by and quietly ask for a sweetened beverage or juice to be served for use as an additional treatment until the meal is served.

How can I help?
Try not to judge how someone is caring for their diabetes based solely on their actions . . . you may not know all the facts and misjudge a situation.

The next time you see your coworker ripping into a sugar packet, don't accuse her. Instead, ask her if she's feeling okay. If she's quietly trying to treat a low, she may appreciate your support and help getting the attention of a waiter to either bring her something to drink (e.g., a regular soft drink, juice, or milk) or check on the status of the meal.

Q. When I picked up my father-in-law at the airport last month, the first thing he asked was, "How soon are we going to be eating supper?" At the time, I got really upset that he was more interested in food than meeting his family. Looking back, though, could he have been feeling hypoglycemic and just didn't tell us?

A. When people ask the question, "When are we going to eat?" there is usually a reason behind it. However, the reason a person with diabetes asks it can be different from why someone without diabetes would. So, without directly asking him why he wants to know when you'll be eating, don't jump to conclusions. Travel is notorious for disrupting schedules and delaying meals. This is especially true if crossing time zones and if there were plane delays. The facts are simple: people with diabetes feel best when they are able to eat at regularly scheduled times.

So, depending upon how long his plane ride was and when his last meal was, your father-in-law could well have been worried about hypoglycemia. (Not a fun thing to have happen when first arriving to meet family and friends.) If meals were not served on his plane and he didn't bring any food along, he may have been trying to decide if he would need to stop somewhere in the airport or nearby to have a quick snack. Because he asked "how soon" will we be eating instead of "what" will we be eating, it's reasonable to suspect he was concerned about hypoglycemia.

The next time he visits, plan ahead and be prepared to have something with you (in your purse, pocket, or in the car) that he could use for a snack if he's running low. Anticipate that he may ask you this question. If he does, just ask him calmly if he's feeling low or needs to eat soon. Should he answer "yes," then offer him a quick snack if it will be a while before the next family meal. If he answers "no," then he can clarify for you his interest in asking. Maybe he wants to treat everyone for supper! By not jumping to conclusions but anticipating his needs and openly communicating with him, you'll feel better prepared to enjoy his next visit.

How can I help? Encourage friends or family members with diabetes to carry medical identification—a medical alert necklace, bracelet, or wallet card—that indicates they have diabetes. In times of emergencies, it'll help rescue teams quickly know how to best help them receive the treatment and care they need.

Q. My wife, who has diabetes, is pregnant. If she becomes hypoglycemic, will it harm the baby?

A. Within a pregnant woman's body, blood and glucose travel across the placenta to feed the growing fetus. If a mother's blood glucose level is high, the baby's blood glucose level will rise. However, because the baby has a brand-new pancreas that works well (unlike the mother's), it can produce sufficient insulin to store the glucose away in cells and regulate its blood glucose level. This is why children born to women with untreated gestational diabetes often grow to weigh more than nine pounds!

When a mother has low blood glucose levels, however, the fetus is not affected in the same way. If the blood feeding the fetus is low in glucose, the fetus can self-correct its glucose level to keep it within a normal range. However during a low, if a mother were to fall or injure herself, that could harm the fetus.

To promote a healthy pregnancy outcome, women with any type of diabetes should strive to keep their blood glucose levels as close to normal as possible. Doctors may even recommend striving for a a target range of 60–100 mg/dl. Because this range puts them closer to the level where hypoglycemia occurs, it's not unusual for them to experience more mild episodes of hypoglycemia than usual. But by knowing this, they can take precautions to catch and treat lows promptly.

Q. I teach second grade and have a student with diabetes in my class. Is there anything I can do to help him prevent having an insulin reaction in class?

A. As a teacher, you play a unique role in the care and health of your students, especially those with diabetes. If you're afraid of his diabetes or ignore the fact that he has special needs, you can make it hard for him to excel and successfully cope with his diabetes. However, by taking the time to learn about his diabetes and how he treats it, your caring and supportive attitude will be appreciated by him and his parents.

Sometimes children with diabetes feel different from their classmates who do not have a medical disease and are called "normal." With his parents and his permission and help, you can help his classmates understand what diabetes is. By realizing what he has to do to care for his diabetes (take shots and test his blood), some kids may consider him brave instead of different. Some may even envy the "cool" or "neat" meter he uses to test his blood. By understanding why he keeps candy in his desk and eats it if his glucose level is low, they can help him successfully cope growing up with diabetes.

Because hypoglycemia is most likely to occur before lunch periods and during gym class (if it's before lunch or at the end of the school day), it's important that he eats his prescribed meals and snacks at consistent times. Schedule a conference with his parents to learn how his diabetes is treated and how you can best support him. Work with your school nurse to learn what you can do to help him self-treat a reaction quickly in the classroom instead of having to escort him to the nurse's office first, which will delay treatment. Find out if you can keep an emergency kit in your classroom containing glucose tablets or fast-absorbing carbohydrate that he'll have easy access to if he notices his blood glucose level getting low.

After a hypoglycemic episode, remember that he may experience difficulty concentrating for a while. If his low happened while he was taking a test, ask him if he had difficulty completing the test because of his blood glucose level. If he did, offer him the chance to retake the test later in the day or during his recess when he's feeling back to normal.

If you offer your students treats as prizes for academic success, realize that sweets are a prize he may not be able to enjoy. He may not be able to eat birthday treats and holiday candy like the other students. Talk with his parents or guardians to find out what kind of nonfood or low-caloric treats he can have instead. For example, nonfood rewards could include stickers, ribbons, books, tickets to a local movie theater, or baseball cards (with a stick of sugar-free gum).

Q. Sometimes I lie awake at night watching my wife sleep, for fear she may have an insulin reaction and I won't be able to help her. However, my fear is keeping me from sleeping. What can I do to stop worrying?

A. Hypoglycemia can happen at night while someone is sleeping. When people have good diabetes control and can sense when a low is coming on, most will wake up on their own.

Their symptoms at night are much the same as during the day when they're awake, although they may feel their low as part of a nightmare. If your wife has difficulty sensing when her glucose level is dropping, you may wake up first and spot it because she'll become sweaty, toss around, or cry out in her sleep while having a dream. If this happens, wake her up and help her test and treat the low.

Each time she has a nighttime low, encourage her to reflect back to the previous day and identify any possible cause for the low. Often nocturnal reactions are caused by:

- eating less than usual at supper
- skipping or eating a smaller bedtime snack than usual
- exercising more strenuously than usual in the evening (e.g., dancing, walking, yard work, shoveling snow, or playing sports)
- changes in medication or insulin dose

To help you get a good night's sleep and prevent her from having lows at night, your wife should work with her diabetes educator or health care provider to review her diabetes treatment program. If she is having frequent lows, they may ask her to check her blood glucose levels more frequently or even test halfway through the night (e.g., around 2:00–3:00 A.M.) to help determine if her medications, insulin, or diet needs to be modified. Most lows at night can be prevented.

CHAPTER 3

Preparing
Healthy Meals

My brother-in-law was just diagnosed with diabetes.
What can I serve for supper when he and his family visit
this weekend? Can he drink coffee or flavored soft drinks?
Do I need to buy special food for him?

When hosting a dinner party, you may experience a wide range of emotions as you prepare for the special event. Feelings of excitement, nervous energy, worry, and fear can all intermix within you as you anticipate the event. One minute you feel excited to have the chance to visit with friends or family, while the next you're afraid the meal you prepare won't be done on time or taste quite like you hoped it would. Because you're reading this chapter, you may have experienced some of these same feelings the first time you prepared a meal for someone with diabetes.

Whether you're a novice or experienced cook, it's common to feel a little nervous at first, preparing for someone you care about who has diabetes. Often we can work ourselves up with needless worry. If this is how you're feeling, don't panic. Relax. Preparing meals for someone with diabetes isn't hard if you treat it the same way you'd prepare to take an exam. First, you'll need to study a little on the subject—you can do it by reading this chapter—and then apply what you learned when you prepare the meal. Before you know it, you'll be cooking up a storm!

In this chapter you'll learn what people with diabetes are advised to eat, what "exchanges" and "carbohydrate counting" are, and how to modify meals to make them lower in fat and sodium. Plus, you'll learn how to plan menus and identify the different types of sugar found naturally in foods. So sit back and take a deep breath to relax. You may be pleasantly surprised at how easy meal planning can be.

To start you on your way, complete the short quiz below to see how much you may already know about the diet for diabetes.

Nutrition Quiz for Diabetes 101

Directions: Circle the letter of the response that best answers each question below.

1. The diet for diabetes is one where someone:
   A. can't eat any sugar, candy, or sweets.
   B. can't eat meat or high-fat foods.
   C. eats only sugar-free, fat-free, and taste-free foods.
   D. eats meals at consistent times in consistent amounts.

2. If someone with diabetes ate roast beef, potatoes with gravy, carrots, and fresh fruit salad and drank a glass of milk for dinner, which three foods will raise her blood glucose level the most?
   A. roast beef, potatoes, and gravy
   B. potatoes, carrots, and gravy
   C. roast beef, carrots, and milk
   D. potatoes, fresh fruit, and milk

3. Can a person with diabetes eat birthday cake?
   A. Yes—if she makes sure no one sees her eating it.
   B. Yes—if she cuts back on eating other foods at her meal to compensate.
   C. No—eating sweets is not allowed on her diet.
   D. No—cake will cause her to have an insulin reaction.

4. What are carbohydrates?

   A. Carbohydrates are the liquids that remain in the stomach after food is eaten.

   B. Carbohydrates are nutrients in food that give the body energy and consist of starch, sugar, and fiber.

   C. Carbohydrates are the minerals in food that help make our bones strong.

   D. Carbohydrates are water molecules that attach to saturated fat.

5. Which of the following is not a form of sugar?

   A. corn syrup

   B. sour cream

   C. fructose

   D. molasses

6. Which of the following beverages does a person with diabetes need to be careful drinking?

   A. lemonade

   B. unflavored iced tea

   C. diet cola

   D. coffee

Results: Check your responses against the answers located at the bottom of this page. Count up how many responses you had correct. If you were able to answer all the questions correctly, congratulations! You've got a good grasp already of the role nutrition plays in the treatment of diabetes. As you read this chapter, you can focus on polishing your skills with meal planning. If, however, you weren't able to answer all the questions correctly or struggled to answer them, don't panic or feel bad—the quiz was just a way for you to assess how much you know about nutrition. If you keep reading, by the end of this chapter you'll be able to plan meals like a pro!

[Answers: 1—**D**, 2—**D**, 3—**B**, 4—**B**, 5—**B**, and 6—**A**]

As you start learning about the diet for diabetes, you may find it at first a little technical-sounding and a bit overwhelming. If you've never had to think about what you eat before, you may even feel as though meal planning takes all the fun out of the simple act of eating. Don't fret . . . it's a normal reaction. Learning about nutrition for the first time is like wearing a new pair of sunglasses. At first things may look different or unusual, but that's because you're looking at them in a whole new way through different-colored lenses. With a little time and practice, though, your eyes start to readjust, and things look more normal. Similarly, over time and with practice, the diet for diabetes becomes more normal as you settle into a new routine (meal pattern). You may even be pleasantly amazed to learn about the effect nutrition has on the body and how people with diabetes use food to help control their disease.

Q. What is a diabetic diet?

A. When someone uses the term "diabetic diet," they are referring to the way or manner in which a person with diabetes eats. The diet for treating diabetes is based on the concept of eating a variety of healthy foods at consistent times in consistent amounts throughout each day. This helps the body control and prevent the blood glucose level from swinging too high or low.

What's ironic is that in the past the term "diabetic diet" used to refer to a very restricted way of eating. However, today the diet is so healthy and full of common sense that it's not even called a diabetic diet anymore. In fact, the diet mirrors the dietary guidelines health experts recommend all Americans follow. These guidelines are to:

- eat a variety of foods
- eat three meals a day along with healthy snacks (as needed)
- choose foods low in fat and high in fiber
- avoid excess amounts of sodium (salt)
- drink alcohol in moderation, if you do so

Q. I remember hearing that people with diabetes can't eat certain foods, especially sugar. Can you explain what foods they need to avoid?

A. The diet for diabetes in years past used to be a very strict, limited way of eating. Up until the early 1900s, people with diabetes were not allowed to eat bread, fruit, or meat or even drink milk, because it was felt that those foods raised their blood glucose level too high. Only by fasting (not eating) were they able to achieve some sort of blood glucose control. Needless to say, this starvation-type diet was neither popular nor healthy to follow. People who followed it progressively lost weight and eventually died from both their diabetes and malnutrition.

When insulin was discovered in the early 1920s, the diet began to change. Finally, people with diabetes were allowed to eat more food as there was an effective medical way to treat diabetes. Diabetes was no longer a death sentence for those who had it. Instead, through better nutrition and blood glucose control, they were able to regain lost weight and their health.

In the 1920s, the early diets for diabetes in the post-insulin era consisted mainly of eating fat, some meat, and a few vegetables. The diet was high in fat (70%) and low in protein (10%) and carbohydrate (20% total calories). People were allowed to have only a little fruit, milk, grains, or starchy vegetables (e.g., potatoes or corn). Sweets and all forms of sugar were strictly forbidden. The diet was neither fun to eat, easy to follow, nor totally nutritious. It was designed to be purely functional (see the table on page 77) .

Over the next seventy years, the diet became more realistic, easier to follow, and healthier as the balance between carbohydrate, protein, and fat calories was adjusted as a result of advances in research, technology, new types of insulin, and medications. Over time, the carbohydrate content of the diet was increased to provide roughly half of the total calories a person consumed in a day. Instead of trying to control diabetes by restricting or adjusting the food eaten, diabetes can be controlled through eating a consistent amount of healthy food each day and adjusting, instead, the medication dose someone takes. This became possible as new ways to measure and control glucose became available.

Today, the diet for diabetes is one that allows a person to eat a variety of foods and promotes healthy eating habits for life.

How the Diet for Diabetes Has Changed over the Past 75 Years				
Diet for Diabetes	1925	1950	1975	2000
Calories from fat	70%	40%	35%	Less than 30%
Calories from protein	10%	20%	20%	10–20%
Calories from carbohydrate	20%	40%	45%	50–60%
Sample dinner (600 calories)	¾ cup cooked pasta in cream sauce 1 1-ounce meatball ¾ cup buttered carrots Coffee with ½ cup cream	1 cup cooked pasta in ½ cup tomato sauce 1½ 1-ounce meatballs ½ cup buttered carrots ½ slice garlic toast 1 cup whole milk	1 cup cooked pasta in ½ cup tomato sauce 1½ 1-ounce meatballs 2 cups lettuce salad with 2 tbsp. low-fat salad dressing 1 slice garlic toast ½ cup 2% milk	1½ cup cooked pasta in ¾ cup chunky tomato sauce 2 1-ounce meatballs 1 cup lettuce salad with 2 tbsp. low-fat salad dressing ½ cup fresh fruit ½ cup skim milk

There are two keys to how the diet for diabetes works. The first key is to not skip meals, but, rather, eat three meals a day at roughly the same time each day. This means not eating simply one or two large meals during a day (e.g., skipping breakfast and possibly lunch and then eating a large supper and evening snack) or delaying meals.

The reason for eating on a regular basis is that the body works and feels the best when it is given food to burn as energy throughout the day. It's like a bonfire. For a bonfire to keep burning strong, it needs fuel (wood). Unless the bonfire is periodically fed wood for energy, it will begin to smolder (die out). Like a bonfire, the human body feels the best when it is given fuel (food) throughout the day; otherwise, it begins to starve and lose energy. When a person has diabetes, he already has a problem with how his system uses food for energy. Therefore, it's important for him to work with his body and feed it on a regular basis to feel his best. (This is good advice for people without diabetes, too!)

So instead of skipping meals or eating meals spaced far apart, the diet for diabetes attempts to space meals typically four to six hours apart during the day. This helps the body regulate its blood glucose level and ensure that food (fuel) is always available for the body to burn as energy. If meals need to be spaced further apart, snacks may be eaten between meals.

The second key to the diet for diabetes is to eat roughly the same amount and type of food at meals and snacks from day to day. When the amount of food (especially carbohydrate) at meals is consistent, it's easiest to keep blood glucose levels steady. In reality, what this means is that someone should avoid eating a large vegetable salad for lunch one day and two slices of deep-dish pizza the next day, because the nutrient composition of the two meals is very different. Thus, the effect of the two meals will be different on blood glucose levels. To

> *How can I help?* If you know someone with diabetes who avoids eating fruit or vegetables because of his diabetes, encourage him to see a registered dietitian or diabetes educator to review his meal plan and show him how to work these foods into his diet.

balance out the nutritional content of the two meals, a person would need to have soup and crackers or a bagel with the salad. Keeping the meals balanced and consistent from day to day helps doctors determine the right insulin or diabetes medication dose a person needs and ensures that it works most effectively.

Q. If people with diabetes can eat whatever food they want, why do they have to follow a specific diet?

A. Healthy people with diabetes who have good control over their diabetes can eat most types of food. While this allows them to eat many formerly forbidden foods (e.g., fruit, birthday cake, or cereals), they still need to watch their portion sizes—how much food they eat—and when they eat. In order to keep the size of their meals the same from day to day, if they decide to occasionally eat something high in calories, fat, or sugar—like a cookie—they have to watch their portion size and substitute it for something else in their meal plan. By planning ahead, they learn to watch how much they eat of a certain food and adjust their intake accordingly. For example, if they choose to eat a cookie, they may need to cut back on how much bread or fruit they have at a meal.

Now, don't interpret this as meaning that they don't need to watch out for what they eat. They still have a serious, chronic disease to manage. The diet for diabetes does not encourage people to eat large amounts of high-fat, -calorie, or -sugar foods. That wouldn't be healthy for them or anyone else. Instead, the dietary guidelines recognize that it needs to be realistic and enjoyable if people are to follow it their entire life. Thus, the diet allows people the ability to include some sweets, if they want them, in their diet. For example, it gives them the option of having a cookie or piece of birthday cake with a meal like anyone else, and removes the guilt they may have felt eating something sweet to celebrate a special holiday.

Just as in life there are always catches, there is a catch to the diet for diabetes. If someone with diabetes needs to lose weight to manage her diabetes, then she needs to closely limit how often she eats high-fat and -calorie foods—the same as someone overweight without diabetes would need to. Also, if someone with diabetes has additional medical conditions that require diet treatment, she may need to follow other dietary restrictions. For example, those with high blood pressure should avoid foods high in salt, while those with heart disease need to watch out for cholesterol and saturated fat in their diet. Those with kidney problems may need to watch out for meat and high-potassium foods (for example,

How can I help? Do you know what foods your friend with diabetes eats or needs to watch out for? If you don't, ask!

bananas and tomatoes). Consequently, the diet that people follow to treat their diabetes and promote overall health can vary slightly from person to person, depending upon any other needs they have.

Q. My brother-in-law was just told by his doctor that he has diabetes. Is there anything I need to keep in mind when planning meals this weekend when he and my sister visit?

A. When you're entertaining guests and aren't sure what to serve because someone has diabetes or some other medical condition, there are two tips to help take the guesswork out of meal planning. First, if you know the person well, call him up and ask him what he can eat as well as whether there are any foods he doesn't eat. He'll be flattered that you care enough about him to ask about his welfare and needs. Once you have an idea of what kinds of food you can serve, the next tip is to plan your meals like you would for feeding a small child.

How does this work? Well, picture what it's like caring for an active five-year-old. While a child can be active playing, he will stop when he feels hungry. When he's hungry, he wants to eat right away. Because of his small stomach and body size, he requires scheduled meals and snacks through the day. But as we grew, our eating habits changed from how we ate as children. Our schedules get busy, and we learn to delay our meals and hold off our hunger in order to get projects done. We learn the habit of eating meals on the run—grabbing high-calorie convenience foods and drinks—instead of sitting down to eat relaxing, healthful meals. When a person has diabetes, they need to get back to eating healthy foods on a regular basis, like small children.

How can this help with planning meals? It helps when we recognize that while children need to eat at scheduled times, sometimes adults need to, too. So, when entertaining guests with diabetes, start your menu planning process by first identifying the times when you will be serving meals and snacks. Be a considerate hostess. Remember to:

■ *Let everyone know in advance what you're planning to serve for meals.* Not only will this allow you the chance to find out if they will like eating what you make, but it lets them know what to expect. The person with diabetes will appreciate this courtesy.

■ *Find out when your guests usually eat their meals.* Find out if they need between-meal snacks. Then, whenever possible, try to accommodate their needs by serving meals near those times. Doing this will help the person with diabetes know how to plan ahead about when to take their medications and insulin, if they use any.

■ *Plan to serve three meals during each day.* Space them four to five hours apart if you're not sure when your guests eat or if they work an evening/night shift, but visit during the day.

■ *Try not to delay serving meals from the times you set, once you announce them.* Remember that while you can delay your meals, it's hard for people with diabetes and small children to do so.

■ *Offer guests the option of a light snack if meals are unexpectedly delayed or are further than five to six hours apart.* This will help tide them over until the meal is ready.

■ *Keep a bowl of fresh fruit on the kitchen table (or counter) and cut-up fresh vegetables on hand for guests to munch on between meals or in the evening.* This allows children, adults, and the person with diabetes easy access to a healthy snack to curb hunger and to help keep blood glucose levels from getting too low if you've had an active day playing.

Q. Do I need to make special food for people who have diabetes?

A. In most instances, you won't need to prepare special foods for people with diabetes, as they are usually able to eat the same healthy meals you prepare for yourself and your family. However, if you're not sure how healthy your meals are, that's a different matter, and you may need to cook different foods from what you're used to preparing when they visit. Take the quiz on page 82 to assess your eating style.

How Healthily Do I Eat?

Directions: Check the box under the response that best describes how each statement applies to your current eating style.

I eat 3 meals a day.

☐ Never   ☐ Sometimes   ☐ Most times   ☐ Always

I eat at least 5 servings of fruit and vegetables a day.

☐ Never   ☐ Sometimes   ☐ Most times   ☐ Always

If I eat potatoes or pasta, I don't eat corn or peas at the same meal.

☐ Never   ☐ Sometimes   ☐ Most times   ☐ Always

When I eat meat, poultry, or fish I keep my portion to no more than 3–4 ounces.

☐ Never   ☐ Sometimes   ☐ Most times   ☐ Always

I eat food high in calcium every day (e.g., milk, soy milk, cheese, yogurt, or calcium-fortified foods).

☐ Never   ☐ Sometimes   ☐ Most times   ☐ Always

I bake, grill, or roast food instead of frying it.

☐ Never   ☐ Sometimes   ☐ Most times   ☐ Always

I avoid cooking with butter, half-and-half, cream, lard, bacon drippings, or sour cream.

☐ Never   ☐ Sometimes   ☐ Most times   ☐ Always

I don't add salt to my food.

☐ Never   ☐ Sometimes   ☐ Most times   ☐ Always

I eat more grains, fruit, and vegetables than I do meat, fat, and sweets.

☐ Never   ☐ Sometimes   ☐ Most times   ☐ Always

I don't eat dessert with my meals.

☐ Never   ☐ Sometimes   ☐ Most times   ☐ Always

Results

- If you answered "most times" or "always" to all of the statements above, pat yourself on the shoulder. You have many healthy diet habits to be proud of and will have little trouble preparing meals for people with diabetes.

- If you answered "sometimes" or "never" to most of the statements above, your diet includes foods that may not be easy for people with diabetes to eat because they are high in fat, calories, and possibly sodium. At first you may find it challenging to prepare meals for someone with diabetes. But with practice, you will find that it's not hard, and you may even enjoy eating your meals like theirs for the health benefits you can receive from eating nutritiously.

Q. How can I plan well-balanced meals that are healthy?

A. To help with meal planning, use the Food Guide Pyramid on page 84 as a way to ensure that your meals contain a variety of healthy foods. The Food Guide Pyramid assigns food into six food groups called the starch, fruit, vegetable, dairy or milk, meat/meat substitute, and fat/sweet groups. By picking and choosing foods from each food group, you can build well-balanced meals in the blink of an eye. Here's how the pyramid works.

Just as a pyramid is built upon a wide, solid foundation, the foundation of a well-balanced diet is eating plenty of grains and starches to provide sufficient carbohydrate for the body to make glucose from. Foods such as bread, rice, pasta, cereal, and starchy vegetables (i.e., peas, corn, and potatoes) make up the starch group and provide most of the carbohydrate our bodies need for energy. As a pyramid rises, it gets smaller toward its top; so do the amounts of food a person needs from the food groups that go on top of the pyramid's starch base. The second level of the food pyramid is comprised of fruits and vegetables, which provide the essential vitamins and minerals our bodies need to form strong bones, healthy cells, maintain a strong immune system, and prevent malnutrition. As the food pyramid continues upward, the third level consists of foods rich in protein—dairy, meat, poultry, fish, nuts, legumes, and meat substitutes (e.g., tofu). Consuming adequate protein is important, as protein is used by the body to repair and build cells, maintain the acid-base balance of blood and regulation of body fluids, and transport molecules throughout the body. The fourth and last level of the food pyramid allows for some fats and sweets to top off a well-balanced diet for flavor and fun. This level includes condiments, desserts, and beverages we may have (besides milk or juice) with a meal.

To create a nutritious, well-balanced meal, include at least one item from each food group. Offer more starches, fruits, and vegetables than meats, fats, and sweets, so your meal will be pyramid-shaped and include a variety of nutrients. Be careful. If you find yourself serving meals that omit food groups, your meal will become top-heavy, causing your food pyramid to become off-balance. This can happen if you serve more chips, dip, and

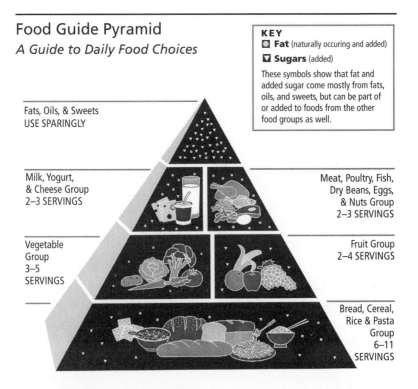

Food Guide Pyramid
A Guide to Daily Food Choices

KEY
▢ **Fat** (naturally occuring and added)
▼ **Sugars** (added)

These symbols show that fat and added sugar come mostly from fats, oils, and sweets, but can be part of or added to foods from the other food groups as well.

Fats, Oils, & Sweets
USE SPARINGLY

Milk, Yogurt,
& Cheese Group
2–3 SERVINGS

Meat, Poultry, Fish,
Dry Beans, Eggs,
& Nuts Group
2–3 SERVINGS

Vegetable
Group
3–5
SERVINGS

Fruit Group
2–4 SERVINGS

Bread, Cereal,
Rice & Pasta
Group
6–11
SERVINGS

cookies than fruits and vegetables. Off-balance meals (where the way you eat doesn't match the food pyramid) often lack the necessary nutrients, vitamins, and minerals that a person needs to stay healthy.

> **How can I help?**
> Try to include at least one food item from each food group when you plan your meals.

When cooking for someone with diabetes, meals need to be well-balanced. Serving off-balance meals makes it hard for a person with diabetes to find foods he can eat that fit his diet and keep his blood glucose level under control.

To help you plan healthy meals, complete the activity below. Use the space provided to try your hand at writing a balanced menu using the food pyramid as your guide. After you complete one menu, try planning a few more or even a full week's worth of menus—breakfast, lunch, and supper. Be adventurous and creative.

Creating Balanced Menus

Imagine that you have guests coming over tonight for dinner. Using the food pyramid on page 86 as your guide, follow the directions below to create a nutritious, balanced meal on page 87.

1. Select what you would like for your main entrée by picking at least one item rich in protein from the meat/meat substitutes food group. Write the entrée you selected on the top line of the sample menu located on page 87.
2. Pick one or two foods from the grains/starches food group that complement your entrée. Add them to your menu.
3. Pick at least one food from the vegetables food group to add color, fiber, and vitamins to your meal. Add it to your menu.
4. Pick one food from the fruits group that you could serve at your meal as either an appetizer, side dish, salad, or natural dessert. Add the fruit you selected to your menu.

Food Group: Fats		Food Group: Condiments	
Butter	Mayonnaise	Jam/Jelly	Horseradish
Bacon	Olive oil	Syrup	sauce
Gravy	Salad dressing	Catsup	Taco sauce
Margarine	Sour cream	Mustard	Vinegar

Food Group: Dairy

Kefir
Milk, low-fat
Pudding, sugar-free, low-fat
Yogurt, low-fat, sugar-free

Food Group: Meat and Meat Substitutes

Cheese, low-fat
Chicken, poultry
Eggs
Fish
Lean cuts of meat: beef, pork, lamb, or game meats
Peanut butter, nuts
Tempeh
Tofu
Legumes (also counts as a starch)

Food Group: Vegetables	
Bean sprouts	Mushrooms
Broccoli	Okra
Carrots	Spinach
Cauliflower	Tomatoes
Green beans	Water
Lettuce	chestnuts

Food Group: Grains/Starches		Food Group: Fruit
Bagels	Plantain	Apples
Bread, buns, or rolls	Squash	Bananas
Cereal, hot or cold	Potatoes	Berries
Corn	Rice	Fruit cocktail
Crackers	Rice cakes	Fruit juices
Noodles/pasta	Tortilla	Grapefruit
Pancakes	Pumpkins	Grapes
Peas	Yams	Melon

5. Identify the condiments you'll need at your meal to complete the menu, choosing from the fats/sweets–condiments food group. Add these to your menu.

6. Decide what beverages you can serve with the meal. *Note:* Offering milk or noncaloric beverages as options is always a good idea when entertaining people with diabetes.

Example: *off-balanced menu*	*Example:* *well-balanced menu*
Fried chicken with gravy	Baked chicken
Fried potatoes	Garlic mashed potatoes
Creamed corn	Warm dinner roll
Flaky biscuits with honey	Steamed green beans
Lemonade	Fresh fruit salad
	Light margarine
	Milk or iced tea with lemon

Create Your Own Menu

Meat/meat substitute	=	_____
Starch choice #1	=	_____
Starch choice #2	=	_____
Vegetable	=	_____
Fruit	=	_____
Condiments	=	_____
Beverages	=	_____

Q. How do lasagna and chili fit into the food guide pyramid and menus I write?

A. Foods like lasagna, casseroles, pizza, sandwiches, and tacos are examples of what dietitians call *combination foods.* Combination foods are entrée or main dish items that consist of two or more food groups.

To determine how combination foods fit into the food pyramid, you need to consider what main ingredients make up the food item in question. That will help you gauge what food groups are in the combination food. For example, consider a slice of pizza. The pizza crust is a type of bread, so it would contribute a starch serving. The tomato sauce and any onions, green peppers, or vegetables would count as vegetable servings. If there is cheese and/or meat on the pizza, it would add a meat and possibly a fat serving. Thus, a slice of pizza could contain servings from the starch, vegetable, meat, and fat food groups. To balance out the pizza and make a well-balanced meal, all you have to do is add a serving of fruit for dessert and a glass of milk to drink.

Using Combination Foods		
Food Item		*Typically Consists of These Food Groups*
Slice of pizza, deluxe	=	Starch, vegetable, meat, fat
Taco	=	Starch, vegetable, meat, fat
Lasagna	=	Starch, vegetable, meat, fat
Tuna noodle casserole	=	Starch, meat, fat
Chili	=	Starch, meat, vegetable

Q. Where can I find sample menus I can follow if I don't want to create my own?

A. Sample menus can be helpful when first learning to cook for someone with diabetes. They're like a picture next to a cookbook recipe—the picture gives you an idea of how the recipe should look after it's made so you can assess how well the food turned out. In the same way, sample menus are useful in knowing what a well-balanced menu looks like. Sample menus are also useful to help create grocery shopping lists to ensure that you have the necessary ingredients to make a meal.

On page 89 is a sample menu to give you a picture of what you could serve. In the back of this book (Appendix C), there are more sample menus you can follow to help you with meal planning. For additional sample menus, see the recommended reading list (Appendix A) also at the end of the book.

How can I help?
As a host/hostess, your responsibility is to offer a selection of healthy foods. It's your guest's responsibility to know how much food he needs to eat.

Sample Menu

Breakfast
Scrambled eggs (use a liquid egg substitute for a low-fat
alternative)
Toasted whole wheat bread with low-fat margarine and
low-sugar jam (fruit preserve)
Fresh fruit
Low-fat milk
Coffee or tea

Lunch
Vegetable soup
Turkey sandwich (whole wheat bread with sliced turkey,
fresh vegetable relishes, and spicy mustard)
Soda or oyster crackers
Fresh fruit cup
Milk, coffee, or a sugar-free soft drink

Supper
Baked fish with lemon
Baked potato with low-fat margarine
Steamed vegetables
Tossed lettuce salad with light vinaigrette, served on the side
Angel food cake topped with fresh berries and a dollop of
nondairy whipped topping
Low-fat milk, coffee, or a sugar-free soft drink

Evening Snack
Air popped popcorn

Q. I've heard my mother talk about "exchange lists." What are they?

A. Exchange lists are a method some people with diabetes use to help with meal planning. Based on the six food groups of the

Food Guide Pyramid, foods in each group are assigned a specific portion size based upon their nutrient value—how much carbo-hydrate, protein, and fat are in each food item. Some foods were reassigned to different food groups based on their nutrient com-position, so like foods are grouped together. For example, while peas are technically a vegetable, they are high in carbohydrate and act upon a person's blood glucose level like a starch serving (slice of bread). Thus, peas are called a starchy vegetable and reassigned to the starch food group.

People with diabetes use exchange lists in conjunction with a prescribed meal that acts as a menu template to help prepare meals that are consistent from day to day. A meal plan shows how many servings (portions) from each food group one should eat at each meal. It is designed to work in sync with diabetes pills and/or insulin to keep blood glucose levels regulated. What's nice about using the exchange lists with a meal plan instead of just using the Food Guide Pyramid for menu planning is that exchange lists promote food portion consistency while still allow-ing meal flexibility. With flexibility, a person is less apt to feel as if she's in a rut eating only the same foods day in and day out.

At first, using exchange lists can seem overwhelming. It requires learning which foods are in each food group, measuring food portions, and planning menus in advance. It's like learning a new language where you first need to learn the alphabet (food portions) before you can put words and sentences together (meals). By investing a few hours in practicing the system and measuring food portions, most people find it's not as compli-cated as it first appears. They can become able to eyeball portion sizes whether dining at home or out. Thus, using the exchange lists helps them feel more in control of their diet and diabetes.

If someone you know with diabetes is unsure of how to use the exchange lists or dislikes the meal plan she has, encourage her to talk with a registered dietitian to obtain a meal plan that allows foods she likes to eat and fits her lifestyle. Meal plans work best when they are tailored to meet the unique needs of each person and not the other way around.

To help you understand how exchange lists work, pretend you are preparing breakfast for a friend with diabetes. Imagine that your friend told you that he likes to eat toast, cold cereal, and a banana for breakfast. If he ate a small bowl of corn flakes with a cup of milk and ½ sliced banana on top and a slice of toast on the side, this would equal two starch portions, a dairy/milk portion, and a fruit portion (see Sample Breakfast Meal below).

Now imagine that one morning your friend announces he wants only toast instead of cereal for breakfast, he could exchange his cereal portion for another slice of toast. As long as he exchanges one portion in the starch group for a different starch item, his blood glucose level should remain steady when his meter readings are compared from one day to another. Thus, exchanging food items within a food group is one way to use the exchange system to add variety to meals.

Sample Breakfast Meal

1 slice bread = 1 starch exchange portion

¾ cup corn flakes = 1 starch exchange portion

1 cup milk = 1 milk exchange portion

½ banana = 1 fruit exchange portion

Now pretend that one morning your friend decides he wants waffles instead of toast for breakfast. That's possible, too! Within each food exchange group, there are many foods he can exchange (see the list below). For example, within the starch food group, he could exchange his two slices of toast for two waffles.

Examples of One Starch Exchange Portion	
1 slice bread	1 corn or flour tortilla, 6–7" diameter
½ cup hot cereal	
½ English muffin	¾ cup corn flakes cereal
bagel, 1 ounce	1 waffle, 4½" square

Another way the exchange lists can be used is to exchange portions between certain food groups. Because the fruit, dairy/milk, and starch food groups contain similar amounts of carbohydrate (roughly 15 grams), for variety at meals people can exchange food portions between these three food groups. For example, if your friend wanted to eat a whole banana at breakfast, he could exchange one of his starch (waffle or toast) portions for another fruit portion. The only food groups that can't be exchanged between are the meat/meat substitute, fat, and vegetable food groups, which contain little carbohydrate.

Q. I've heard that some meal plans allow free foods. What are these?

A. The term "free foods" is used to describe foods and beverages that contain less than 20 calories or 5 grams of carbohydrate per serving. Because their calorie content is so low, a single serving of a free food will have little overall effect on someone's blood glucose level. Thus, the serving doesn't have to be accounted for in their meal plan, it's free (unless they eat multiple servings). Within a meal plan, people with diabetes should avoid eating more than 60 free food calories a day. What is eaten is best tolerated when spread throughout each day. If someone decides to eat all their free food calories at once, the food should be worked into their meal as a food group choice instead of as a free food choice so their blood glucose level isn't affected.

Free Foods/Condiments (less than 20 calories per serving)	
broth (consommé)	mustard
catsup	nondairy creamers (liquid or powder)
fat-free cream cheese	
fat-free salad dressing	nondairy whipped topping (regular or light)
horseradish	
lemon juice	peppers, jalapeño
lime juice	salsa

sugar-free gelatin	sugar substitutes (e.g.,
sugar-free gum	Equal, Sweet One,
taco sauce	Splenda, Sprinkle Sweet)

Free Beverages

coffee	iced tea, sugar-free
tea	soft drinks, sugar-free
flavored drink mixes, sugar-free	or diet
	mineral water

Q. I heard my friend with diabetes talk about "carbohydrate counting." What is that?

A. Once people with diabetes learn to use food exchanges, they often advance to a more sophisticated version of meal planning called "carbohydrate counting." While still based on the Food Guide Pyramid and exchange lists, this method goes one step further in striving to keep the carbohydrate content of meals as consistent as possible while allowing more flexibility in meal planning. The carbohydrate counting approach is based on the fact that there are three food groups naturally high in carbohydrate—the starch, fruit, and dairy/milk groups. Within a meal plan, these food groups are combined to form a new and bigger group called "carbohydrate choices." This merging is possible because each serving of starch, fruit, and milk consist of roughly 15 grams of carbohydrate. So if a meal normally included two starch, one fruit, and one milk portions, this would now equal four carbohydrate choices. Through keeping the number of carbohydrate choices consistent at each meal, people with diabetes can mix and match between the three food groups however they please.

The carbohydrate counting method easily allows a person with diabetes to incorporate new foods into his diet by calculating portion sizes based on a food's carbohydrate, protein, and fat content. This allows him to occasionally fit a sweet into his diet, which wasn't encouraged just a few years ago. For instance, if your friend wanted to have a piece of birthday cake with frosting, he could eat the cake (two carbohydrate choices) in place of two servings of either fruit, starch, or milk that he would normally have had at his meal.

The carbohydrate counting method can be very helpful to people who need to use insulin. Some can adjust the amount of insulin they take to compensate for eating more or less carbohydrate choices at a meal. For best diabetes and weight control, it's important when using the carbohydrate counting method to not forget to eat consistent amounts of meat, fat, and vegetables at meals. While these foods have less of an effect on blood glucose levels than carbohydrate choices, they can still affect diabetes control and promote weight gain, if not watched.

Q. How can I tell how much carbohydrate is in a food item?

A. Knowing how much carbohydrate is in a food item is easy if you read food labels. On food items, manufacturers are required to list the amount of total carbohydrate (and other nutrients) per serving of each food item. The information is listed on the nutrition facts panel of the food label (see page 95).

Q. My husband has diabetes and heart disease, which require that he avoid eating high-fat foods. How can I cook low-fat meals for him?

A. Food high in fat, especially saturated (animal) fat, which contains cholesterol, can contribute to atherosclerosis (hardening of the blood arteries) by depositing a fatty buildup (plaque) on artery walls. If plaque starts to harden and clog the arteries, it increases one's risk for having high blood pressure, a heart attack, or a stroke.

The trick to preparing heart-healthy meals is to first check the ingredients you're using to make your meals. To reduce the amount of fat and cholesterol in food, use lower-fat ingredients in place of traditional ones high in saturated fat. For instance,

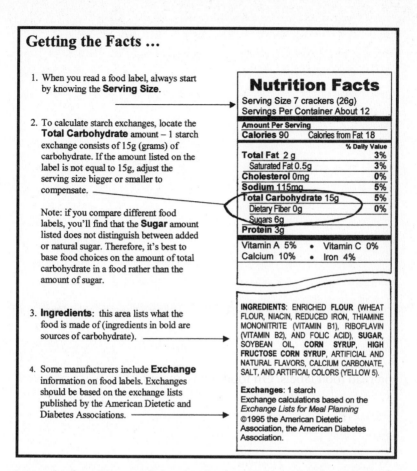

Getting the Facts ...

1. When you read a food label, always start by knowing the **Serving Size**.

2. To calculate starch exchanges, locate the **Total Carbohydrate** amount – 1 starch exchange consists of 15g (grams) of carbohydrate. If the amount listed on the label is not equal to 15g, adjust the serving size bigger or smaller to compensate.

   Note: if you compare different food labels, you'll find that the **Sugar** amount listed does not distinguish between added or natural sugar. Therefore, it's best to base food choices on the amount of total carbohydrate in a food rather than the amount of sugar.

3. **Ingredients**: this area lists what the food is made of (ingredients in bold are sources of carbohydrate).

4. Some manufacturers include **Exchange** information on food labels. Exchanges should be based on the exchange lists published by the American Dietetic and Diabetes Associations.

Nutrition Facts

Serving Size 7 crackers (26g)
Servings Per Container About 12

Amount Per Serving

Calories 90   Calories from Fat 18

	% Daily Value
Total Fat 2 g	3%
Saturated Fat 0.5g	3%
Cholesterol 0mg	0%
Sodium 115mg	5%
Total Carbohydrate 15g	5%
Dietary Fiber 0g	0%
Sugars 6g	
Protein 3g	

Vitamin A 5%	•	Vitamin C 0%
Calcium 10%	•	Iron 4%

INGREDIENTS: ENRICHED **FLOUR** (WHEAT FLOUR, NIACIN, REDUCED IRON, THIAMINE MONONITRITE (VITAMIN B1), RIBOFLAVIN (VITAMIN B2), AND FOLIC ACID), **SUGAR,** SOYBEAN OIL, **CORN SYRUP, HIGH FRUCTOSE CORN SYRUP**, ARTIFICIAL AND NATURAL FLAVORS, CALCIUM CARBONATE, SALT, AND ARTIFICAL COLORS (YELLOW 5).

Exchanges: 1 starch
Exchange calculations based on the
Exchange Lists for Meal Planning
©1995 the American Dietetic
Association, the American Diabetes
Association.

instead of cooking with butter, lard, or bacon drippings, which are high in saturated fat, switch to using canola, olive, corn, soybean, or peanut oils. These are monounsaturated fats and contain no cholesterol. Try margarine made from 100 percent oil instead of butter when cooking, and reduced-fat soft spread margarine at the table to flavor and top foods. Use lean cuts of meat instead of prime cuts, which are heavily marbled in fat.

You can further reduce the amount of fat in foods by using low-fat cooking methods. Instead of deep-frying in oil and sautéing foods in butter, broil, bake, grill, roast, microwave, or steam food. For example, instead of frying chicken or potatoes, try baking or grilling them. Avoid adding high-fat cream and cheese sauces to food; instead, experiment with using herbs and spices to flavor foods in a more natural way. Before adding fat to cooking pans, assess if you really need to add it. Often the new nonstick cookware sold today needs little if any fat to coat the cookware to prevent food from sticking, unlike cast-iron and aluminum pots and pans.

Here are some ways to experiment cooking with less fat.

Low-Fat Low-Cholesterol Ingredient Switching

If a Recipe Calls For	*Switch to:*
Butter	Margarine
Whole milk	Low-fat or no-fat milk
Whole egg	2 egg whites or ¼ cup liquid egg substitute
1 cup vegetable shortening	¾ cup canola or vegetable oil shortening
Vegetable oil (for baking)	Replace some of the oil with applesauce, fruit pureé, or plain nonfat yogurt
Sour cream	Nonfat sour cream or plain nonfat yogurt
Heavy cream	Evaporated skim milk
Cream cheese	Light or low/no-fat cream cheese
Whipped cream	Light nondairy whipped topping
Ricotta cheese	Light or low-fat ricotta cheese
Cottage cheese	Low-, no-fat cottage cheese

Low-Fat Cooking Tips

- Use cooking methods that add little or no fat to food (e.g., broiling, grilling, baking, stir-frying) instead of deep-fat frying.
- Use lean cuts of meat and trim off visible fat before cooking.
- Skim off the fat from chilled soups and stews before reheating or serving.

After you finish preparing your meal, don't forget about the fat that can be added to food at the table. Those watching their fat intake need to avoid using high-fat condiments that add extra calories to food prepared in a healthy low-fat manner. Watch out for serving special mayonnaise sauces with hamburgers and sandwiches, creamy dressings with salads, and sour cream and butter on top of baked potatoes. To keep foods low in fat, always serve sauces, gravies, and dressings in separate dishes (on the side) to allow everyone to decide for themselves if they want to use a condiment or not.

When selecting low-fat condiments to serve guests, check food labels to make sure that the items are lower in both total fat and calories. Sometimes low-fat table toppers (condiments) have extra carbohydrate added to them, which, if used in large amounts, could affect someone's blood glucose control.

Tasty Low-Fat Table Toppers	
catsup	salad dressings, light
flavored light cream cheese	or nonfat
spreads	salsa
horseradish sauce	spicy mustard
hot sauce	whipped or light
light vinaigrette	margarine
mayonnaise, light or nonfat	yogurt, plain, nonfat
salad dressing, light or nonfat	

Q. My husband has high blood pressure. He's supposed to follow a low-sodium diet, but he thinks the food I cook without salt is "blah." How can I get him to follow his diet and quit using a salt shaker?

A. Sodium is a chemical that exists naturally in the food we eat in varying amounts. Our bodies need sodium to help regulate body fluids, conduct nerve impulses, and control muscle contractions. But while our bodies need some sodium, sometimes we consume too much of it. Because sodium attracts and retains fluid, for people who have high blood pressure a high-sodium diet can make it hard for the body to regulate its fluid balance. This can put stress on the heart. The most common source of sodium in our diet is table salt (sodium chloride). Other sources of sodium include foods that are pickled (or preserved in brine), cured meats, soy sauce, and processed foods, which can contain a variety of sodium compounds.

The diet for treating high blood pressure is one low in sodium (salt). However, this doesn't mean *no* salt. Remember, we need some sodium for normal body functions.

Because your husband has gotten used to salting his food, he's learned to like the taste of salt. If you catch him salting his food before he tastes it—whether it's at home or when dining out—it's a sure sign that he likes the taste of salt. So when he tastes food you prepare with less salt and says it tastes "blah," it's because his taste buds have become so used to the salt that they have a hard time picking up on other flavors in the food.

While you can't change your husband and force him to give up his salt shaker, you can make sure he understands how the sodium in salt affects his blood pressure and how salt is a learned taste—a habit—that he's developed, probably over many years. For him to break his habit of using a salt shaker, recognize it will take a lot of hard work and effort on his part. However, with your help you can help him see that there are alternatives to using a salt shaker—spices!

Once your husband decides he's ready to try cutting back on salt, have him replace his salt shaker with a black peppercorn grinder to enhance the flavor of his food. If he doesn't like pepper, he can use any other spice he likes that doesn't contain high levels of sodium. For example, if he likes spicy foods he could try tabasco sauce, horseradish, jalapeño peppers, lemon pepper, or garlic. As he stops using the salt shaker, remind him that food naturally contains sodium, so he's not totally giving up salt—he's just not adding extra to his food anymore. For the first couple of weeks without a salt shaker, he may regard food as tasting bland or boring. That's expected. But if he keeps with it, over the course of a month his taste buds will readjust and soon he'll be enjoying the many natural and subtle flavors in food. He may be surprised to learn how pleasant food and other spices can be when they're not overwhelmed by salt. You'll know he's successfully made the switch when someday, when dining out, he tastes something high in sodium he used to like and is turned off because it's too salty and makes him thirsty.

While your husband works on not using a salt shaker, you can help him watch out for sodium in his diet by helping him learn what foods he needs to avoid or use only in small amounts on an occasional basis. When planning menus, avoid food and ingredients that either taste salty, sound salty, or look salty, for example, ham, bacon, pickles, sauerkraut, and salted snack foods. Avoid using high-sodium condiments such as soy sauce, teriyaki sauce, and garlic or onion salt. Instead, use lower-sodium versions of the sauces, spice powders, or fresh herbs. Offer foods that are lightly seasoned and allow him and others you may prepare meals for to add more spices or pepper to suit their taste. This way, you allow everyone to season their food to meet their own needs and desires, and your husband won't feel singled out as having to eat differently from everyone else.

For fun, you may enjoy experimenting with new spices to season the food you make. If you like spicy foods, try rubbing pepper, garlic, or other spices on meat before grilling them. If you like blackened or Cajun grilled meats, chances are you may have been eating foods low in salt without realizing it. Many ethnic foods use spices other than salt to boost their flavors.

If you want to try using more spices, here are some ideas on how to get started. Know that there is no right or wrong way to use or combine herbs and spices—it's a matter of personal taste. Strive to have herbs accent the natural flavor of food rather than creating one strong herb flavor. Then the only decision you will need to make is whether you want to use fresh, dried, or powdered herbs and spices. If you use dried herbs, you'll find that 1 tablespoon of fresh chopped herbs has a taste that is equal to 1 teaspoon of dried or ¼ of a teaspoon of powdered or ground

---

Did you know . . . dried herbs and spices can lose their flavor if they are not stored correctly. Always store spices and dried herbs in airtight containers to retain freshness. If you're using spices that are a couple of years old, get new ones! You'll be amazed at how much more flavorful they are.

---

herbs (dried herbs have a more intense flavor). To get the most flavor from your herbs, add them to food when you are almost done cooking, as many lose some flavor when cooked for long periods of time.

IF COOKING	FLAVORINGS TO TRY
Beef	Basil, chili powder, dill, garlic, mushrooms, mustard, onions, oregano, pepper (red, white, or black)
Poultry	Curry, garlic, ginger, parsley, paprika, sage, tarragon, thyme, sesame seeds
Fish	Basil, bay leaf, cayenne, celery seed, curry, dill, lemon, mint
Pork	Caraway seed, cinnamon, cloves, Dijon mustard, garlic, onion, oregano, sage
Vegetables	Anise, cilantro, dill, lemon, mixed whole spice, pepper, nutmeg, parsley, rosemary, sesame seed

Q. My aunt has diabetes and problems with her kidneys. I think she has to watch out for meat and potassium in her diet. What food can I cook for her when she visits me over the holidays?

A. The kidneys play an important role maintaining the body's fluid balance, regulating how much sodium, potassium, calcium, and other nutrients are in the body, and removing creatinine (a by-product of protein when it's broken down in the body) from the blood. If your aunt has decreased kidney (renal) function, she needs to be careful how much she eats of certain foods so she doesn't overtax her kidneys. What foods she needs to watch out for depends upon how well her kidneys are working.

People with mild kidney problems often need to limit the amount of meat (or high-protein foods) and sodium they eat. As kidney function decreases, they may also need to watch out for potassium, calcium, phosphorus, and how much fluid they have each day.

Instead, offer moderate-sized portions of meat roughly the size of a deck of cards or an audiocassette tape (roughly 3 ounces cooked meat). You may also consider serving a near meatless meal occasionally; for example, serve a cold pasta salad with vegetables and a taste of tuna or shrimp along with a steaming bowl of old-fashioned vegetable barley soup.

Because you're not sure what foods your aunt needs to avoid or how well her kidneys work, it's best to ask her what foods she normally eats and avoids. This is the quickest and safest way to learn what she can eat when she visits you. If she watches out for sodium, refer to the question above for ways to cook food with less salt. If she watches out for protein, avoid serving large portions of meat, poultry, or fish.

Should your aunt need to watch out for potassium and/or calcium in her diet, here are some quick tips to help you out.

To Cut Back on Potassium

- Try using pasta, rice, or couscous as side dishes instead of potatoes.

- Avoid using vegetables such as tomatoes, corn, broccoli, mushrooms, okra, parsnips, and spinach, as they contain high amounts of potassium. Instead, use lettuce, turnips, green pepper, and small amounts of carrots, cucumber, onion, or green beans.

- Avoid using fruit such as oranges, bananas, melons, strawberries, kiwi, and figs. Instead, use apples, blueberries, cranberries, pears, and pineapples.

- When serving pasta, use pestos, a roux, or cream-based sauces instead of tomato-based sauces.

To Cut Back on Calcium

- Limit the use of dairy products (milk, cheese, and yogurt) in recipes.
- Avoid serving salmon or sardines which have bones.
- Avoid serving calcium-fortified products such as soy milk, tofu, and some orange juices, bread, and rice.
- Avoid collards, spinach, and great northern beans.

It's interesting to note that people who need to restrict their protein intake often need to increase their fat and carbohydrate intake. While this sounds contrary to the usual diet for diabetes, it's necessary for those with kidney problems. The reason for this goes back to the fact that there are three main nutrients that provide calories—carbohydrate, protein, and fat. If protein is restricted to prevent further kidney problems, then the calories the person normally would have consumed from protein need to be replaced with either added carbohydrate or fat. Consequently, people with both diabetes and kidney failure may be prescribed a diet that intentionally has them eating a certain number of sweets and sweetened beverages in order to consume enough calories to maintain their weight and energy level.

Q. I'm confused by what I've heard about diabetes while watching television and talking to relatives. First I heard fruit and sugar were bad to eat—now I learn it's okay. Why are there so many mixed messages?

A. Unfortunately, there are many myths floating around about diabetes and the way to treat it. To understand why, you need to remember that the way diabetes is treated has changed over the past few years. Much of the confusion is due to the fact that outdated information is still being passed around by word of mouth and promoted in books printed before 1994, which are still being sold and are in public libraries. Books printed before 1994 will not contain information from the Diabetes Control and Complications Trial, the United Kingdom Prospective Diabetes Study, or other landmark studies recently published that have changed how diabetes is treated. Therefore, we need to get the good news out that there are new ways to treat and control diabetes in the new millennium! Here are six nutrition myths still floating around that are not true.

Myth #1: Since fruit is a natural food, it's okay for people with diabetes to eat it anytime they want to.

Fact: A sugar by any name—fructose, sucrose, or lactose—is still a carbohydrate. Whether it comes from fruit, bread, milk, or honey, carbohydrate provides calories and will break down into glucose in the body for energy. One form may just be a little quicker than another (seconds versus minutes). For best glucose control, fruit and juice should not be considered "free foods" that can be eaten in unlimited amounts whenever desired. Instead, fruit should be worked into their meal plan the same as bread or milk is.

> *Did you know . . .*
> *it's not so much the type but the amount of carbohydrate in the diet that needs to be consistent.*

Myth #2: People with diabetes can't eat anything that tastes good.

Fact: This myth makes little sense, as it literally implies that if people with diabetes can't eat good food, then they can only eat bad-tasting food. But what is good- or bad-tasting food? If you ask different people, some will say that good food is food that is healthy to eat. Bad food, on the other hand, is high in calories, fat, and sugar and low in vitamins and minerals (e.g., candy bars, sweets, and some snack chips). Were this myth true, it would literally mean that people with diabetes can't eat good (i.e., healthy) foods but only eat bad foods such as candy and sweets! But we all know that a candy diet is not healthy for anyone, let alone someone with diabetes.

If you interpreted the myth to mean that people with diabetes can't eat food that literally tastes good, that also doesn't make sense. Why? Because taste is a matter of personal opinion. What tastes good to one person may not to another. Some may say that good food is a traditional home-cooked meal (like meat loaf and baked potatoes), while others may say that good food is a donut, a hot fudge sundae, or liver and onions. Ethnic foods such as enchiladas, fried bread, gyros, or pizza are often thought to be tasty. But, so can watermelon on a hot day or chili on a cold one. So, the bottom line is that food is really neither good nor bad. Instead, food is food. It's our reaction to it and our eating habits that imply whether a food is healthy or tasty.

Communication activity
The next time you hear someone say, "I wish good food wasn't bad to eat," ask him to explain what he means. Ask him the following questions and find out what he believes about food. You may be surprised at what you learn.

- What is good food?
- What is healthy food?
- How does good food taste?
- How does bad food taste?
- Can healthy food taste good?

Myth #3: People with diabetes shouldn't eat food that has more than 3–5 grams of sugar in it per serving.

Fact: It's true that in the past, people with diabetes were often advised to avoid foods that had more than 3 grams of sugar per serving. But that was based on using the old food labels. Today, this rule no longer works well, since food labels were revised in the mid-1990s. Now the amount of sugar listed on the "Nutrition Facts" food label represents the combined amount of natural and added sugar in a food. Because the label doesn't differentiate between how much of these sugars are in a food item, the rule to limit foods with more than 3–5 grams of sugar per serving doesn't work anymore.

Check it out. The next time you're in the kitchen, look at the food label on a carton of plain milk. On the label, you'll find that one cup of milk has roughly 11 grams of sugar in it! If you followed the myth, you would have to stop drinking milk or putting it on your breakfast cereal, as it contains too much sugar. However, plain milk does not contain added sugar—the sugar listed on the food label represents the natural sugar (lactose) in milk. Because nutritionists expect lactose to be in milk, they recommend that people with diabetes use the "Total Carbohydrate" information on food labels instead of "sugars" when deciding how a food item can fit into one's diet. The total carbohydrate amount represents all the sugar, starch, and fiber in a food, making it a better indicator of how the food will affect blood glucose levels.

Myth #4: If a food is dietetic or sugar-free, it's okay for someone with diabetes to eat it whenever they want to.

Fact: The bottom line is this: the terms "diet" or "dietetic" on a food label do not mean "diabetic." These types of foods are not free for the person with diabetes to eat whenever they want unless they fit the definition of a free food mentioned earlier.

Prior to 1990, manufacturers could print terms such as "dietetic" and "light" on their products without the terms meaning the same thing from one product to another. Something called "light" could mean lighter in color than the original product or lighter in calories or sodium. Terms such as "sugar-free" implied that a food contained no sugar (table sugar, or sucrose), but consumers didn't realize that these same foods could contain other forms of sugar (e.g., honey) and still be called "sugar-free." Consequently, this was misleading to many people, with or without diabetes.

Some people with diabetes purchase foods called "sugar-free" or "dietetic" thinking that they are free foods in their diet. However, this often isn't the case. For example, a few years back a candy company made sugar-free peanut butter cups, which were labeled as "sugar-free" and suitable for people with diabetes. Unfortunately, some people with diabetes misunderstood this to mean they were a free food and ate the candy in unlimited amounts. This resulted in them having poorly controlled diabetes and gaining weight. They didn't know how to work the candy into their diet.

To set the record straight and clear up some of the confusion about what food label terms meant, the Food and Drug Administration (FDA) published definitions for many nutrition words and health claims, including sugar-free and no-added-sugar. Companies can no longer call food sugar-free if it contains a form of sugar—products have to fit the legal definition or be penalized by law. Consequently throughout the 1990s, food companies have redesigned their food labels to satisfy the legal definitions. Here's what a couple of the new sugar terms mean:

- *Sugar-free* means that a food contains less than 0.5 g natural or added sugar per serving (e.g., sugar-free gelatin).

- *No-added-sugar or without added sugar* means that no sugar or sugar-containing foods were added to a food while it was being made. However, the food may contain other types of carbohydrate and contain the same total calories as its original version (e.g., no-added-sugar apple pie).

- *Unsweetened or no-added-sweeteners* means sugar was not added to a food during processing (e.g., unsweetened orange juice).

When reading food labels, be an informed shopper and know whether you're getting what you think you're buying. If you are thinking about buying something that's reduced in sugar (such as cookies, candy, or pie at a restaurant), ask to see its "Nutrition Facts" information. Check to see if it contains any carbohydrate (see list on page 107). Then, check the ingredient panel to see if the product contains any forms of sugar. Remember, it's the amount of total carbohydrate (sugar, starch, and fiber combined) in a food that is the best indicator for how the food will fit into one's diet.

Myth #5: High-protein, very low-carbohydrate diets are a healthy way to treat diabetes and promote long-term weight loss.

Fact: Popular diets come and go over the years. The high-protein, low-carbohydrate diet is one such diet that cycles through

Other Names for Sugar Found on Food Labels

- cane (sugar cane)
- corn or maple syrup
- corn sweetener
- dextrose or dextrin
- disaccharide
- erythritol
- fructose (fruit sugar)
- high-fructose corn syrup
- honey
- hydrogenated saccharides
- hydrogenated starch hydrolysate (HSH)
- invert sugar
- isomalt
- lactose (milk sugar)
- maltose (malt sugar)
- maltodextrin
- mannitol
- molasses
- natural sweeteners
- sorbitol
- xylitol

almost every generation. While different variations of this diet theme exist, it usually promises to improve blood glucose levels, promote weight loss, and sometimes even increase muscle. However, it doesn't hold up to its promise on a long-term basis. If you want to build biceps and gain strength, muscle conditioning exercises are more effective than eating lots of meat. These diets aren't a lasting solution for weight control, either, as they're hard to follow on any long-term basis and are not always nutritionally sound. In fact, for the person with diabetes who has heart or kidney problems, it can be potentially dangerous!

Can people lose weight and lower their blood glucose level with these types of diets? Initially, yes. However, the weight loss first achieved can often be attributed to either a simple reduction in total calories consumed (i.e., eating less) or a loss of body fluid (i.e., water). Most of the calories being cut out are from consuming less sweets, sugars, and alcohol. Because weight loss occurs through consuming less total calories, blood glucose, cholesterol, and even blood pressure levels can improve.

But are these diets the miracle answer to weight loss and diabetes? No, the diets often encourage people to avoid foods which contain carbohydrate—blaming carbohydrate as the cause for obesity and poor diabetes control. While carbohydrate does affect blood glucose levels, to avoid eating them also means staying away from milk, potatoes, rice, and juice. That often leaves a diet that allows maybe a slice or two of bread; lots of meat, poultry, and fish; and high-fat condiments!

When diets promote avoiding food groups and foster a fear of eating, it's a sign that they are unrealistic and do not promote long-term health. People who follow these diets are at risk for gaining the weight back, as few are able to stay on them for their entire life because they are so restrictive. If they stop following the diet and go back to their old eating habits, most regain their weight plus a few extra pounds. This promotes the myth that carbohydrate-rich foods cause weight gain! It's not the carbohydrates that cause weight gain, it's eating more calories from carbohydrate, protein, fat, and alcohol—combined—than what your body needs for energy.

Another problem with very low-carbohydrate diets is that they often caution against eating vegetables and fruits, which are high in vitamins and minerals. The diets miss the fact that low-carbohydrate and very-low-calorie diets are often lacking in many of the vitamins and nutrients that promote heart health. A diet low in fruits and vegetables can put one at risk for high blood pressure and certain types of cancer. Taking supplements to put back the vitamins and minerals that are missing may help, but it isn't the answer—eating a nutritionally balanced diet is.

A healthy diet should consist of a variety of foods, eaten in moderation. The diet should be balanced between carbohydrate, protein, and fat to promote overall health and wellness, and feel satisfying enough to maintain for a lifetime.

Myth #6: Diabetic food and cookies taste blah and are unappealing.

Fact: If you have ever had diabetic cookies made from recipes in old cookbooks, it's true that many were unappealing. Years ago, diabetic recipes were modified to remove as much sugar from them as possible—especially in desserts. However, when cooks did this they didn't always adapt the recipes to use a different tenderizing agent or more spices to flavor the food. Thus, the recipes often resulted in food that tasted blah, looked blah, and had a texture vastly different from that of the original recipe.

Today's recipes for diabetic desserts and meals are very tasty. By using more spices, sugar substitutes, and other ingredients to compensate for sugar, new diabetic recipes are popular with people of all ages and types (with and without diabetes). Because they are often lower in fat and calories than traditional recipes, they are popular with people with heart disease and those who are trying to lose weight.

Q. What foods should I keep on hand for my granddaughter to eat when she visits me? She has type 1 diabetes.

A. If your granddaughter is only going to be eating just one or two meals with you, you don't really need to purchase special foods for her. However, if she visits often or is going to visit for an extended amount of time, you may wish to have a few foods on hand that she enjoys and can look forward to eating. Here are examples of foods you may want to have on hand for meals and snacks. But before you go out and buy any, check with your granddaughter and her parents to learn what she likes (so you don't buy something she doesn't like that just sits in your cupboard).

> *Beverages:* flavored mineral water, diet soda, sugar-free soft drinks, no-added-sugar cocoa
>
> *Condiments:* sugar substitute, light or simply fruit jam/jelly, sugar-free syrup, light salad dressings, soft-spread margarine
>
> *Cupboard Staples:* animal crackers, biscotti, crispbreads, ginger snaps, graham crackers (regular, chocolate, or cinnamon), low-fat muffin mixes, matzo, melba toast, popcorn,

pretzels, rice cakes, sugar-free gelatin, sugar-free pudding mix, unsweetened canned fruit, vanilla wafers

Q. Can I serve wine or a beer to someone who has diabetes?

A. While many people enjoy a glass of wine or alcohol with a meal, people with diabetes need to be cautious drinking it. Why? Well, besides having calories, alcohol is a toxin to our body. After we consume it, our body tries to excrete (get rid of) it from our systems as soon as possible. As a result, the body's ability to control its blood glucose level is affected in the process. In people with good diabetes control, a glass of an alcoholic drink tends to lower a person's blood glucose level. However, this effect can happen hours after a person drinks it, longer if the alcohol is consumed on an empty stomach. Because of this, people with diabetes who take insulin or diabetes pills are at risk for hypoglycemia when they drink alcohol.

This doesn't mean that people with diabetes can never have a glass of wine or a beer. If their diabetes is under good control, people with diabetes can usually tolerate having one to two drinks with a meal a couple of times a week. The best time to have alcohol is with a meal—either just before, during, or after. They should avoid drinking on an empty stomach between meals.

For those people who are overweight and control their diabetes without insulin or medication, they need to consider that alcohol contains calories. To avoid weight gain, they should work the glass of alcohol into their diet to account for the calories it provides. What this means is that they may need to cut back on the amount of fat they consume in their meal, thereby exchanging the fat calories for alcohol calories. Some may also need to avoid using alcohol if they are pregnant, using other medications that interact with alcohol, or have a history of alcohol abuse.

If you serve alcohol at a meal or party, start by offering everyone a choice of beverages—some with alcohol and some without. This polite gesture allows people to decline or accept alcohol. When you serve alcohol, choose drinks that do not contain added sugar. Here are some ideas on what you could serve:

Try Serving	Avoid Serving
Wine	Sweet wines
Champagne	Wine coolers (made with syrup or sweeteners)
Light beer	
Distilled liquor (1 shot = 1½ ounces) mixed with ice or sugar-free flavored soft drinks	Liqueurs
	Cordials
	Mixes with sugar or syrups (e.g., flavored margarita mixes)

Q. At our local bakery, they make and sell no-added-sugar pies and candies. Are these okay for my husband to eat?

A. Large bakeries, manufacturers, and restaurant chains that make health claims about their food are required, under the FDA food labeling laws, to be able to show consumers the nutritional information for their food. However, small bakeries, restaurants, and delis are exempt from these rules. Because of this, don't automatically assume that marketing claims on pies and candy will not have an effect on your husband's diabetes unless you can find out what they're made of. If the salesclerk says a pie doesn't contain any sugar, she may be right. Pie crusts don't routinely contain sugar in them. However, they are made from flour or grains, which are a form of carbohydrate. If the pie is filled with fruit and used juice or natural sweeteners instead of sugar, that's also carbohydrate. This also holds true for candy. When a local store claims that something is made without sugar, find out if they mean that white sugar was not used. Find out what the item is made of. Often the no-added-sugar candies contain other forms of sugar and can have just as many calories as the regular item. Thus, besides not always tasting as good as the regular item, specialty products are often higher in price and can still affect blood glucose levels.

This doesn't mean that there aren't some wonderful products being made by some bakeries. There often are. However, it's buyer beware to make sure you are getting what you want when buying sweets.

Think about it . . . Often we've been brought up to include dessert with our meals. But do we really need or want it after a well-cooked meal? If a meal is filling in itself, try finishing it off with a relaxing cup of coffee and pleasant conversation instead. Another option would be to serve a simple fruit cup instead of traditional high-fat and high-calorie cakes, sweets, or ice cream.

Q. Why does my husband sometimes get diarrhea and abdominal gas after eating sugar-free candy?

A. Some sugar-free candies are made from natural sweeteners called sugar alcohols (polyols). Polyols are used in candy, medication, and food because they are extremely sweet and don't provide as many calories as sugar. One such example of a polyol is sorbitol, which is used in items ranging from sugar-free candies and breath mints to cough drops and vitamins. When eaten in large amounts, sorbitol can cause gas, bloating, cramps, and diarrhea. Not quite the effect you'd want if you're sick with a cold and sucking on cough drops.

Typically, it takes around 50 grams of sorbitol to cause diarrhea. However, some people may be sensitive to polyols and react to as little as 5–10 grams. That's the amount of sorbitol in only two to five sugar-free breath mints or pieces of hard candy. Because sorbitol is also found naturally in fruit and fruit juices, that's another source to be aware of.

So if your husband feels gassy or bloated after eating a few pieces of sugar-free candy, he may want to check the ingredient list for sorbitol. If he thinks he may be sensitive to it, he should try finding a different brand of sugar-free candy or limit how much he eats of it.

Q. Are sugar substitutes like aspartame and acesulfame-potassium safe to use? I heard that aspartame isn't good for

people with diabetes and could cause multiple sclerosis.

A. For years, non-caloric sweeteners and sugar substitutes have been used around the world to flavor foods. But before they are allowed in the United States, the FDA requires extensive testing to ensure that sugar substitutes such as aspartame, sucralose, and acesulfame-potassium are safe to use and will not cause health problems. Despite hoaxes and Internet rumors that sweeteners are hazardous for general usage, the following sweeteners have been shown to be safe if used in moderate amounts.

Non-Calorie Sweeteners: Which Is Which?			
Generic Name	Brand Name	Sweetners Compared to Table Sugar	Uses
Acesulfame-potassium	Sweet One	1 packet = 2 tsp. sugar	As a condiment or in baking and cooking
Aspartame	Equal, Nutrasweet Spoonful	1 packet = 2 tsp. sugar, 1 tablet = 1 tsp. sugar	As a condiment or with cooking cold or hot foods (not with baking)
Saccharin	FeatherWeight, Sucaryl, Sugar Twin, Sweet 'N Low	1 packet = 2 tsp. sugar, 1 tablet = 1 tsp. sugar	As a condiment, with baking and cooking, or with canning
Sucralose	Splenda	1 packet = 2 tsp. sugar	As a condiment or with baking or cooking

In 1999, both the American Diabetes Association and the Multiple Sclerosis Foundation assured the public that rumors about the sweeteners causing diseases are false and without merit. Still, a small number of people have reported being sensitive to using some sweeteners. When this is the case, it's recommended that they avoid using the offending sweetener and try a different one. For the future, there are two other sweeteners—alitame and neotame—that are pending FDA approval.

Did you know . . . in 1998, a national consumer survey by the Calorie Control Center reported that over 144 million Americans used low-calorie foods and beverages that are sweetened with sugar substitutes. And this number is on the rise!

CHAPTER 4

Caring During Illness and High Blood Glucose

WHEN MY WIFE GETS THE FLU, SHE USUALLY CAN'T KEEP ANY FOOD DOWN. SHOULD SHE STILL TAKE HER INSULIN IF SHE CAN'T EAT? HOW CAN I HELP HER?

All of us experience illness at one time or another. Maybe it's a summer cold or a winter flu bug. Maybe it's something worse, like an injury or infection. Whatever it is, though, it makes us appreciate having good health and helps us become more sensitive to the needs of others—a friend, family member, or coworker—when they are ill. Tender care from family and friends can bring comfort to those who are ill and help the healing process go a little easier, nicer, and faster. It doesn't have to be much—maybe just a cheery card, a hug or shoulder rub, or a friendly voice to talk to. It's the thought and care that matter.

However, when a person who is ill also has diabetes, you may wonder how you can help him without affecting his blood glucose control. You may wonder what types of food to give him if he can't swallow well due to a sore throat, or can't keep food down due to the flu. This chapter will review the effect illness has on diabetes. It will explain what hyperglycemia and diabetic ketoacidosis are and also offer tips on how to help someone whether near or far away. Let's start with the basics.

Q. How does illness affect blood glucose?

A. When we are sick or have an injury, our bodies cope with the stress of being sick by releasing hormones that help the body fight off infection. This process results in the blood glucose level rising, regardless of whether we have diabetes or not. Normally, the body would self-correct the high glucose level by producing more insulin. However, when someone has diabetes, she isn't able to do this, as she has a problem with either making insulin or using it. This results in her blood glucose level going up and staying up. When blood glucose levels stay above normal, it's called *hyperglycemia*.

Q. What causes hyperglycemia?

A. Hyperglycemia can be caused by a number of reasons. Most often it's due to:

- eating larger meals than usual
- eating more carbohydrate-rich foods than usual
- being less active than usual
- not taking insulin or diabetes pills
- being under severe stress
- having an illness or infection
- taking a new medication for something besides diabetes

Q. Is hyperglycemia dangerous?

A. Hyperglycemia can cause both long- and short-term problems. On the long-term side, when blood glucose levels stay above normal for a long time (months and years), it takes a gradual toll on body cells and tissues, putting people at high risk for diabetes complications such as kidney, eye, and heart disease. The risk they face is like owning a car in Minnesota and never washing it. They may get away with having a dirty car for a few years. But after years of driving in snowy weather without washing off the grime and deicing chemicals used on the roads, the car will start to show signs of rust. To prevent rust and maintain the car's beautiful appearance, a car owner needs to continually care for the car by keeping it regularly washed and waxed.

Like taking good care of a car, having good blood glucose control can help someone with diabetes delay or prevent health complications. Two significant studies in the 1990s proved this. The Diabetes Complications and Control Trial (DCCT) in 1993 showed that people with type 1 diabetes who took aggressive care of their diabetes reduced their risk for developing complications by up to 75 percent. In 1998, the United Kingdom Prospective Diabetes Study (UKPDS) confirmed that good blood glucose control also reduces complications in people with type 2 diabetes, but at lesser rates than seen in the DCCT study. Either way you look at it, the bottom line is that there are long-term risks for developing diabetes complications when glucose levels stay elevated and are not treated, but long-term benefits when it is.

On the short-term side, when blood glucose levels stay high (above 240 mg/dl), it means that the body is having trouble using glucose for energy. This can cause people to feel tired, thirsty, hungry, and have a frequent urge to urinate. When cells aren't able to get the glucose they need from the bloodstream, they turn to the body's stored fat and protein for energy. Unfortunately, when the cells use fat for energy, they also need some insulin around for the process to work effectively. If insulin isn't present, the byproducts of cells using fat for energy (called *ketones*) can start to build up in blood and body tissues. Because ketones are toxic to the body's system, they can cause the body to become acidic.

Q. What happens when the body become acidic from ketones?

A. When ketones build up in the body to a point where blood and tissues become acidic, it's called *ketoacidosis* or *diabetic ketoacidosis* (DKA). When this happens, the body tries to rid the ketones from its system and return the body to a neutral pH level by having the kidneys filter ketones out of the blood and excrete them in urine. The lungs also join in and try to help detoxify the body. They do this by converting ketones into carbon dioxide, which can be exhaled from the body. However, this process causes a person to breathe very rapidly and deeply, and have a fruity odor to the breath. If ketones build up faster than the body can get rid of them, it can lead to severe dehydration, illness, and coma.

Considered a serious complication of diabetes, DKA can develop quickly (within hours to days) and requires prompt emergency medical treatment, often even hospitalization. People with type 1 diabetes are most susceptible to DKA because they lack the ability to make insulin. DKA can develop when glucose levels remain above 300 mg/dl.

The symptoms of DKA are easy to spot once you know what to look for. In addition to the usual symptoms of high blood glucose (see page 19), watch for the symptoms listed below. If the person you know with diabetes becomes ill and shows any of these symptoms, encourage him to check his blood glucose level and for ketones. Promptly call his health care provider for assistance in controlling his blood glucose levels if his blood glucose level is high and he's spilling ketones in his urine.

Symptoms of DKA

- lack of appetite
- stomach pain or nausea
- vomiting
- fever (flushed skin)
- unusually rapid, deep breathing
- fruity breath
- sleepiness
- dry mouth
- dehydration
- low blood pressure
- rapid heart beat
- shock
- coma

People with type 2 diabetes are less likely to experience DKA because they are still able to make insulin. While their bodies may produce ketones as the result of burning fat for energy, they don't produce as much because they are still able to use some glucose for energy. Consequently, their body doesn't become as acidic and they can often tolerate higher blood glucose levels than people with type 1 diabetes. For people with type 2 diabetes, hyperglycemia can develop slowly, over a period of days or weeks. It can creep up on someone when they're sick.

Because people with type 2 diabetes can tolerate higher glucose levels without becoming acidic, they are at risk for developing a condition called *hyperglycemic hyperosmolar nonketotic syndrome* (HHNS). HHNS is often brought on during illness or other medical conditions that affect blood glucose control, such as untreated infections, a stroke, stress, and untreated diabetes. When glucose levels start climbing above 500 mg/dl, the risk for HHNS is high. When HHNS develops, it can result in severe dehydration, which can cause blood to flow poorly throughout the body. When this happens, it can lead to organ failure and death.

Because symptoms of HHNS develop slowly, it's important for people with type 2 diabetes to check their blood glucose level more often when they become ill. When glucose levels remain over 250 mg/dl, they should call their doctor for medical advice. If it is higher than 500 mg/dl, they need urgent medical treatment.

Symptoms of HHNS (in addition to those of hyperglycemia)

- dry or parched mouth
- confusion
- extreme thirst
- warm dry skin, but no sweating
- sleepiness
- disorientation

Did you know . . . *some people can tolerate higher levels of glucose better than others? Often people with type 2 diabetes who don't use insulin or diabetes pills will report that their blood glucose level was over 1,000 mg/dl when their doctor diagnosed them with HHNS. A person with type 1 diabetes wouldn't be able to tolerate such a high level. For this reason, how high someone's blood glucose is doesn't relate well to how serious a DKA or HHNS episode is. Tolerance levels vary per individual. Bottom line: All DKA and HHNS episodes are serious and life-threatening.*

Q. How are DKA and HHNS treated?

A. When DKA and HHNS strike, people with diabetes need the prompt help of their health care provider. Often this will be done in a hospital setting. The first thing that the doctors will do is replace the body fluids lost through dehydration. They will also closely monitor the electrolyte levels (e.g., sodium, potassium, and magnesium) in their blood and replace any that are affected by the dehydration. With the help of insulin, they will gradually lower the blood glucose level back to normal.

How can I help? If someone has hyperglycemia and can't get in to see her doctor right away, encourage her to drink lots of water and avoid being physically active. This can help prevent her blood glucose and ketone levels from going even higher and help her fight off dehydration.

Q. How do people know when they have ketones? Can they test for them?

A. Yes. When blood glucose levels stay above 240 mg/dl, people with diabetes should test for ketones in their urine using urine ketone test strips. To do this, they need to apply some of their urine to a small test strip that has a testing pad (spot) on the end of it. If ketones are present in the urine, the test pad will change color. The test pad can then be matched to a color chart that indicates the amount of ketones present as small, moderate, or large.

How can I help? If someone has type 1 or 2 diabetes and his blood glucose level is over 250 mg/dl and spilling ketones into his urine, encourage him to call his health care provider.

Q. I remember that my father used to test his urine, but I thought that was for testing his glucose level. Do people still test their urine for glucose?

A. Ever since self-monitoring blood glucose testing meters became available, it's not common for people to measure their glucose level by checking their urine. This is because the test doesn't give results as accurately as a meter and can't measure for low glucose levels. The urine test only measures how much glucose the kidneys filtered out of the blood into the urine. It doesn't reflect what someone's current blood glucose level is and can provide false high results if taken after drinking a large glass of orange juice—vitamin C in juice can interfere with the test—or after taking some medications, aspirin, iron, and some vitamin supplements.

However, as a backup to meters, some people keep some urine glucose test strips around for times when they can't use a meter, for instance, when they're traveling someplace where they can't take their meter or their meter battery runs low. In these instances, urine glucose testing gives them a temporary method to make sure that their glucose level doesn't get too high.

Q. When my wife gets the flu she often can't keep any food down. Should she still take her insulin or diabetes pills when she can't eat?

A. Yes. The number one rule for people with diabetes when they're ill is to always keep taking their diabetes pills or insulin. This is because when they are ill, their blood glucose level will go up regardless of whether they eat or not. So despite the fact that she may not be eating much, it's important that she take her medication to help keep the blood glucose level under control. If she doesn't, she runs the risk of developing hyperglycemia and feeling worse. On sick days, she may also need to adjust her dose of insulin to compensate. If she doesn't know how to do this, she should ask her doctor or diabetes educator.

Unfortunately, many people with diabetes forget this rule when they're sick and stop taking their pills or insulin. All too often, they

> *How can I help?*
> *When someone is ill, remind them that they always need to take their diabetes medication even if they don't feel like eating.*

end up needing medical care for hyperglycemia they could have prevented.

Q. When my husband gets a sore throat, he doesn't like to eat. What can I give him to encourage him to eat?

A. Preparing meals for someone who's ill can be challenging and depends on what he can tolerate. Often, this can vary from meal to meal; in the morning, he may want only liquids, but by night he may be ready for solids. In addition, during illness he may lose his appetite and complain that food tastes blander or is less appealing. This can make it extra-challenging for you, as a helper, to find things he will eat.

To make mealtimes easier for you and him, plan ahead for sick days by stocking a variety of convenience foods you can offer if he is unable to eat his usual meal. Things to stock in your cupboard include soup, hot and/or cold cereal, boxed meals, sweetened soft drinks, individual servings of fruit juice, soda, and graham crackers, and regular gelatin or pudding mix. Sometime when he's feeling well, ask him to give you a list of foods he likes to eat when sick. Also, obtain a copy of his meal plan or ask him how many servings from each food group he usually eats at each meal.

Using his meal plan, you can convert his usual meals into sick-day meals. Complete the activity below to learn how.

Creating Meals for Sick Days

Part A.   Calculating Carbohydrate Choices

1. Identify how many servings from each food group the person with diabetes usually eats at each meal. Transfer this information into the column titled "Regular Meal Plan." While you do this, identify to the left of the plan what time of the day he usually eats each meal.

2. Transfer the number of starch, fruit, and milk servings at each meal and snack to the "Carbohydrate Choices" column located

Sick Day Meal Pattern

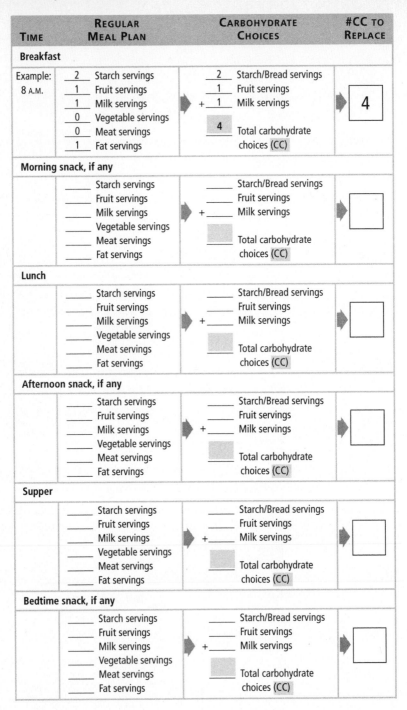

Time	Regular Meal Plan	Carbohydrate Choices	#CC to Replace
Breakfast			
Example: 8 A.M.	2 Starch servings 1 Fruit servings 1 Milk servings 0 Vegetable servings 0 Meat servings 1 Fat servings	2 Starch/Bread servings 1 Fruit servings + 1 Milk servings 4 Total carbohydrate choices (CC)	4
Morning snack, if any			
	___ Starch servings ___ Fruit servings ___ Milk servings ___ Vegetable servings ___ Meat servings ___ Fat servings	___ Starch/Bread servings ___ Fruit servings + ___ Milk servings ___ Total carbohydrate choices (CC)	
Lunch			
	___ Starch servings ___ Fruit servings ___ Milk servings ___ Vegetable servings ___ Meat servings ___ Fat servings	___ Starch/Bread servings ___ Fruit servings + ___ Milk servings ___ Total carbohydrate choices (CC)	
Afternoon snack, if any			
	___ Starch servings ___ Fruit servings ___ Milk servings ___ Vegetable servings ___ Meat servings ___ Fat servings	___ Starch/Bread servings ___ Fruit servings + ___ Milk servings ___ Total carbohydrate choices (CC)	
Supper			
	___ Starch servings ___ Fruit servings ___ Milk servings ___ Vegetable servings ___ Meat servings ___ Fat servings	___ Starch/Bread servings ___ Fruit servings + ___ Milk servings ___ Total carbohydrate choices (CC)	
Bedtime snack, if any			
	___ Starch servings ___ Fruit servings ___ Milk servings ___ Vegetable servings ___ Meat servings ___ Fat servings	___ Starch/Bread servings ___ Fruit servings + ___ Milk servings ___ Total carbohydrate choices (CC)	

to the right of the regular meal plan. After you've transferred the number of servings, add up the servings to determine how many total carbohydrate choices this equals. (*Note:* He doesn't need to replace the meat, vegetable, and fat servings in his meal plan, as they contain little or no carbohydrate.)

3. Transfer the number of starch, fruit, and milk choices he has at a meal into the "Number of CCs to Replace" column. Add the numbers together to determine the number of carbohydrate choices he'll need to replace with sick-day foods and liquids if he is unable to follow his usual meal plan.

Part B   Planning Menus for Sick Days

There are three golden rules to follow when planning sick day meals for people with diabetes. After you have determined how many servings from each food group and carbohydrate choices he usually has at his meal, menu planning is based upon what foods he can tolerate. Follow these rules.

Golden Rule #1: *Before each meal, ask him if he can handle eating regular food and follow his normal meal plan.*

If he can tolerate chewing and swallowing regular foods, offer him foods that are soft-textured and easy to eat, for example: toast, scrambled eggs, hot or cold cereal, soups, casseroles, cottage cheese, soft roast meats, or soft cooked vegetables. Encourage him to drink sugar-free, decaffeinated beverages or water between meals to prevent dehydration.

Golden Rule #2: *If he isn't feeling up to regular foods at a meal, ask him if he could tolerate chewing or swallowing soft foods (solids) or liquids.*

If he is having problems chewing, swallowing, or holding down food, you'll need to substitute the usual number of carbohydrate choices he eats at each meal or snack with sick-day food choices. For example, if he usually has three carbohydrate choices at breakfast, then he would need to replace them with three sick-day food exchange portions. You'll be replacing the regular types of carbohydrate food he has with some regularly sweetened foods and beverages to help provide him with the calories and energy he needs to get well and help keep his blood glucose level under control. Using the worksheet below, you can mix and match foods he can tolerate to create a special sick-day meal just for him.

At each meal or snacktime, you'll need to reassess if he is able to tolerate regular food yet or if he'll need to keep using sick-day food exchanges instead. By assessing his status on a meal-to-meal basis, you'll be able to help encourage him to take in adequate amounts of carbohydrate and calories in order to have the energy to fight off his illness while keeping his diabetes under control. Between meals, encourage him to drink noncaloric, caffeine-free beverages for hydration, for example, sugar-free soft drinks, decaffeinated hot tea, sugar-free gelatin, or Popsicles. A good goal to aim for is to have him try to drink or sip one cup of fluid per hour.

Note: On sick days when someone isn't able to eat much, the most important way to help him is to replace the carbohydrate choices from his meal plan. You don't need to worry about replacing the vegetable, meat, or fat servings, because once he is feeling up to eating solids again, you will be able to work him back into his diet. The key is to keep his carbohydrate intake consistent. While this will make his diet lacking in some nutrients, it will only be for a short time (hopefully, just a meal or two).

Regular (Soft) Foods for Sick Days

Starches	toast, soft breads, soft tortillas, noodles, rice, couscous, cooked or cold cereal, mashed potatoes
Fruit	canned fruits without seeds or skins, applesauce or fruit sauces, soft fruits (e.g., bananas), fruit juice
Vegetables	any soft cooked vegetables, juices, vegetable soup
Meats	eggs (poached, scrambled, omelets), cottage cheese, tender cuts of meat and poultry, fish, creamy peanut butter
Milk/Dairy	cream soups, milk, sugar-free flavored yogurt or pudding

NUMBER OF CCS TO REPLACE	TIME	SICK-DAY REPLACEMENT MEAL

Breakfast

Snack

Lunch

Snack

Supper

Snack

Sick-Day Food Exchanges—Solids
(Each portion equals 1 carbohydrate choice)

1 slice toasted bread

½ toasted bagel, 1 ounce

½ cup cooked cereal

⅓ cup rice or couscous

1 waffle, 4½" square

3 graham cracker squares, 2½"

6 soda crackers

2 rice cakes, 4" round

½ cup applesauce or fruit sauce, unsweetened

½ cup canned fruit, unsweetened

Sick-Day Food Exchanges—Liquids
(Each portion equals 1 carbohydrate choice)

½ cup apple or orange juice

⅓ cup grape juice

½ cup sweetened soft drink

½ cup regular gelatin

½ cup ice cream

⅓ cup frozen yogurt, regular

½ cup frozen yogurt, sugar-free

½ cup sherbet

1 cup soup

1 cup milk

½ cup chocolate milk

½ cup pudding, sugar-free

¼ cup pudding, regular

½ cup custard

⅓ cup yogurt, sweetened with fruit

1 cup yogurt, sugar-free

Golden Rule #3: *If he is unable to keep any food down, ask him if he could sip on liquids.*

It's important on sick days that the person with diabetes doesn't become dehydrated. So if he is able to sip on liquids, try having him sip slowly on sweetened beverages like flavored fruit drinks, sports drinks, or caffeine-free soft drinks. Often people with upset stomachs find soft

> **How can I help?**
> Help plan ahead for sick days by creating sick-day menus that are converted from the usual meal plan to include a variety of solids and liquids.

drinks (e.g., cola) soothing to sip on. A good goal would be for him to try to sip at least one-half to one cup of fluid per hour. If this is too much for him, aim for a couple of sips every fifteen to thirty minutes.

Q. If my son has the flu, at what point should he or I call his doctor for help?

A. If your son gets the flu and continues to throw up or have diarrhea for more than half a day and is unable to keep any food, liquid, or medications down, you or he should contact his health care provider for assistance. They can advise him if he needs to temporarily change an insulin or medication dose and obtain medication to fight off the flu.

Q. When my husband is ill, he loses his appetite and complains that food tastes bland. What can I do to get him to eat?

A. There are a number of ways you can encourage someone to eat if he's lost his appetite or doesn't feel like eating. Here are some tips you can try:

- Suggest different temperature and textured foods to help him find something that appeals to him. For example, ask if something soft, warm, cold, crunchy, or salty would be appealing.

- Experiment with adding spices and herbs to food if it tastes bland to enhance the food's flavor (see page 100). Avoid adding extra salt if his blood pressure control is a concern.

- Plan menus that include a variety of colors. If serving macaroni and cheese and toast, which are mostly white and yellow, add a splash of color to the meal through garnishes and vegetables.

- Assess if the smell of food bothers him. If it does, try cooking foods in the microwave instead of on the stove or in the oven, which emit more odors. Have him stay in a different section of the house while you're cooking so he doesn't smell the food until right before he eats.

- Try cold meal choices like sandwiches, cold pasta salads, cold cereal, cottage cheese, and canned fruit that have little odor.

- Open a window or have him sit outside on a porch if the weather is nice. A little fresh air can help stimulate sluggish appetites.

- Create a pleasant place for him to eat. Try setting a pretty table, playing relaxing music, and promoting pleasant, relaxed conversation while eating. Avoid arguments and having children misbehave at the table.

Q. My wife sucks on cough drops when she has a cold. Is that okay? Could they affect her blood glucose level?

A. Regular cough drops usually contain some form of sugar for sweetness. So, they do have the potential to raise her blood glucose level if eaten in large numbers throughout a day. If they are only used on an occasional basis (one or two during the day) to suppress a cough or soothe a dry mouth, the small amount of sugar in them is probably not enough to have a big effect on her blood glucose control. The benefits of not coughing outweigh the small potential rise in blood glucose levels. However, if cough drops or throat lozenges are used frequently, people with diabetes need to be aware of the effect they can have on glucose control. If this is the case, sugar-free throat lozenges may be a solution. A variety of companies make sugar-free cough drops and lozenges that are well tolerated by people with diabetes if used in small amounts. Be careful, though, as some sugar-free candies and lozenges contain sorbitol, which some people are sensitive to. If they are, they may notice that the sugar-free lozenges

How can I help? You can help encourage someone to eat when she has a poor appetite by creating pleasant meals that include a variety of foods with different textures and tastes.

have a laxative effect if they're used in large amounts over a short period of time. Check with your pharmacist for names of sugar-free cough drops and lozenges.

Q. When my husband was in the hospital, they served him a cookie on his lunch tray! I thought that in hospitals, of all places, they would be careful to not serve sweets to someone with diabetes. Should I have said something to somebody there to tell them about the cookie?

A. Hospital and nursing home meals for people with diabetes have changed, just as the diet for diabetes has changed. This is even reflected in the names hospital meals are being called. Where hospital meals varied from place to place and were called diabetic, calorie-restricted, low sugar, no-added-sugar, or no-concentrated-sweets, they are now serving meals that are consistent in the amount of carbohydrate they contain. By serving the same amount of carbohydrate at meal and snacktimes on a day-to-day basis, doctors and patients are finding that it helps with blood glucose control while allowing more food options. This helps encourage ill patients to eat and regain their health.

Because the length of stay in hospitals is often short, when people are hospitalized they are usually very ill and have poor appetites. Since hospitals can serve meals at set times with consistent portion sizes, it's easy for them to serve meals that are consistent in carbohydrate content. This allows a variety of foods that are nutritious and tempting to eat to be on the hospital menu. Examples include serving soups, casseroles, sandwiches, meat-and-potato or rice meals, and even cookies or a small portion of a dessert.

Encouraging people to eat while they are in the hospital is important, as good nutrition helps them recover from their illness faster. Also, by allowing patients to have a small cookie or dessert occasionally, they report that they are often more satisfied with their meals. By receiving foods similar to what other patients in the hospital receive, they also report feeling less isolated and restricted by their diabetes.

Q. Are there things I should keep on hand in our house in case my husband, who has diabetes, becomes ill?

A. It's a smart idea to plan ahead for sick days so you'll be prepared for any occasion that may arise. This prevents late-night dashes to the local drugstore or supermarket for supplies when you least want to. It also helps prevent having to hunt for items you know you have, but can't find. When planning ahead for illness, consider making an emergency sick-day kit. Use a box or container with handles you can easily store in a closet when your husband feels well, but can pull out on days he feels ill. Consider including the following items in your kit:

- phone numbers and addresses of doctors, nurses, pharmacy, urgent care and emergency centers
- ketone test strips
- extra lancets and blood testing supplies
- thermometer
- acetaminophen
- antidiarrhea and antinausea medicine
- sugar-free throat lozenges, decongestants, antihistamines, and sugar-free cough syrup
- sick-day liquids: regular soda and sweetened fruit drinks
- sick-day foods: regular gelatin and pudding mix, sweetened soft drinks
- sick-day meal plans

After you make your kit, remember to store it someplace that's easy to access. Let everyone in your house know where the kit is located and that any food or beverage in the kit is for sick-day use only. This will help ensure that the food is there when you need it in case someone decides to snack on it. Check the expiration dates for items in the kit periodically, so that you have fresh supplies.

Q. My best friend and neighbor, who has diabetes, has been ill lately. I am wondering how I can help her during this tough time. What can I do to help her?

A. The gift of friendship and caring is a wonderful thing to give to someone when she is ill, whether she has diabetes or not. While it's common in our society to give gifts of candy and sweets, often it's the small activities of time and talent that are most meaningful and appreciated.

If your neighbor has found it hard to do the simple activities of daily living—cleaning, shopping, and cooking—start by asking if you could help her out with one of them. Many times, when people are feeling ill they don't like to ask for help, as they don't want to impose on others. This can be especially true of those who live alone and don't have relatives living nearby. Here are ideas on how you can help:

- Stop by to visit and chat for a few minutes over a cup of coffee or glass of iced tea. Nothing brightens up a day more than a smile and a friendly visit.

- Ask her if she would like you to pick up any books from the local library.

- Ask her if she'd like to take a ride in your car to get out of her house for a few minutes. There's nothing like a change of environment for a few minutes to help make someone housebound perk up and smile.

- Ask if she needs any help with her housework—offer to carry a load of laundry up- or downstairs for her, vacuum a floor, or sweep her front doorstep, porch, or kitchen floor.

- Ask during winter months if she needs help shoveling snow off her sidewalk, driveway, or roof after a storm.

- Offer to help her weed or prune her flower garden if she is unable to get outside.

- Offer to help her with spring and fall housework—raking

leaves, washing windows, shaking out rugs, removing or putting on storm windows and screens.

■ Offer to take her to one of her doctor's appointments if she can't drive herself.

■ Offer to pick up grocery staples for her when you go shopping for your family—pick up a carton of eggs, a quart of milk, fruit or juice, frozen dinners, or fresh produce.

■ Surprise her with the gift of a freshly baked loaf of bread, a fruit basket, flavored coffee beans, homemade soup, or some flowers from your garden.

■ Offer to take her to church if she has difficulty getting there.

Q. My aunt is in a nursing home. What can I bring her as a treat or gift that won't bother her diabetes?

A. Often when people who are in hospitals, extended care facilities, and nursing homes for any length of time, there are times when you'd like to give a gift. Gifts are a way, in our society, in which we often express to another that we care for and appreciate someone.

If you wish to bring a gift, you'll need to consider a couple of things. First, you'll need to know how much space she has in her room. If she is sharing a room with someone else, she may not have enough space for big presents like plants, furniture, or framed pictures. Second, you'll need to know if she has any physical impairment that could prohibit using certain gifts. For example, if she has poor eyesight, large print books or books on audiotapes would be better choices than books with print that may be too small to read. Third, you'll need to know what kind of dietary restrictions she has. If you want to bring food or candy, check with her nurses before you give it to make sure it's okay for her to eat. They will be able to tell you if she should have it or not. If she is ill, the nurses may not want her to eat candy or sweets between meals, as that can make it harder to control her diabetes and promote healing. The nurses may ask if they can save the cookie or piece of birthday cake you bring, until her next mealtime, when it can be worked into her meal plan. That way she can have a treat and good diabetes control, too. If you're looking for creative gift ideas that won't affect her diabetes, consider the following.

Gifts from the Heart—Give the Gift of . . .

- drawings/paintings by children to hang on her wall
- family photos—update your album with a new group photo
- notes from family members describing their favorite memories of her
- balloons to hang at the end of her bed
- fresh flowers in a small vase
- seasonal decorations
- assorted greeting cards and stationery with stamps
- books on audiotapes
- bath powder, perfume, or aftershave
- crossword puzzles or word puzzles
- colorful magazines on a favorite topic
- bright, cheery calendars with colorful pictures
- small portable radio/CD player with headphones
- cassettes or CDs of her favorite music
- new bed jacket or piece of clothing
- inspirational daily calendars

If you live out of state and can't visit in person, consider these ideas if you want to brighten her day.

- Call frequently to say hello and tell her you care, especially on holidays.

- Write letters and include clippings of amusing items from your local newspaper.

- Send audiotapes from children and grandchildren sending greetings, updates on what they did at school, or singing a song they just learned.

- Give her a tape recorder so she can send messages back to her children and grandchildren.

- Send home videos that show what's new at your house and in your neighborhood or her old neighborhood.

- Call and ask for her advice on something she used to do— nothing is nicer than to know you're still needed and respected.

- Mail her a copy of a new book.

CHAPTER 5

Planning Special Occasions with Confidence

I WAS PLANNING ON HAVING MY FAMILY OVER FOR THANKSGIVING DINNER. HOWEVER, MY MOTHER WAS JUST DIAGNOSED WITH DIABETES. CAN SHE EAT A TRADITIONAL HOLIDAY DINNER?

The turkey and stuffing are out of the oven and sounds of laughter fill the air as family members prepare for a holiday meal. The house is full of smells—sage, nutmeg, and pumpkin—that invite diners to gather around tables and share a meal together. Holidays are meant to be special times to look forward to and savor.

However, in our society, holidays often revolve around food, many of which are family favorites that can be high in fat, sugar, and calories. While this usually isn't a problem for most people, it can become a challenge to people with diabetes. In addition, because holidays often include travel, preparing and eating meals at different times of the day, and unplanned events popping up, they can become stressful for both the people planning them and the people with diabetes attending them. This chapter will give you tips and ideas on how to make holidays and celebrations times that are relaxing, fun, and healthy for everyone—including those with diabetes. It will also discuss simple courtesies, or "diabetic etiquette," to keep in mind to make special times less stressful for those with diabetes or others who are watching what they eat. Let's get started.

Q. I invited my entire family to celebrate Thanksgiving at my home this year. However, my brother says holidays are hard for my sister-in-law because she has diabetes. They would rather have everyone eat at their place. Why would holidays be hard for her?

A. While only your sister-in-law can really answer your question, it's possible to hazard a guess about why holiday meals are easier for her at her home. Holidays are steeped in traditions and often include high-calorie, high-fat food and sedentary activities. While some things are loads of fun, others can make it difficult for someone with diabetes to keep control of their blood glucose level and enjoy the special day. Here's why.

When holiday meals include five-courses or so much food you could almost feed an army, it becomes challenging for guests to decide what and how much to eat. Those with diabetes—like your sister-in-law—may can be faced with tempting choice of eating foods that are inappropriate for her diet. If she decides to eat high-calorie foods or sweets, she runs the risk of having elevated blood glucose levels and others asking her if she is cheating on her diet. If she doesn't eat the food, some may ask why she isn't honoring family traditions or encourage her to just enjoy the day and forget about her diabetes. Add to this scenario going to someone's house for dinner (at noon) only to find out that the meal is delayed for one to two hours because an out-of-town guest hasn't arrived or the turkey isn't thoroughly cooked yet. If she's taken her diabetes medication expecting to eat at noon, she runs the risk of hypoglycemia if she doesn't eat. However, this would mean that she would need to start eating before everyone else does. Sometimes it can seem like she's caught in a no-win situation when all she wants to do is enjoy the holiday like everyone else.

While others may forget about someone having diabetes or take it lightly, those with it can't. Diabetes is always with them and always needs to be managed. When people with diabetes decide to avoid eating the holiday foods that are inappropriate for their diet, they may feel sad or isolated. This is because the food becomes a reminder to them that they are different; they can't easily eat what everyone else can without affecting their blood glucose control. A recent survey by the American Diabetes Association revealed that people with diabetes often

How can I help? Instead of making events bigger and grander each year, make gatherings simple and relaxing for all involved.

wished their friends and families planned meals that were appropriate for their diets when they gathered for special occasions. By this, they wished families would consider serving foods lower in fat and that are healthier than some traditional favorite holiday foods. Because of this, some people with diabetes may find it easier to host a gathering so they can control their environment. They can ensure that meals are served on time and contain a variety of food they know they can eat.

To help you identify if your holiday gatherings are easy or hard for people with diabetes to attend, take the quiz below.

Assess the Stress of Your Parties

Directions: Imagine you're hosting a holiday party for close friends and family. As you read each of the questions below, answer with either a "yes," "no," or "unsure" response.

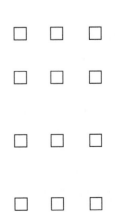

	Yes	No	Unsure
1. Do your guests know ahead of time what kind of food will be served (e.g., a meal vs. snacks)?	☐	☐	☐
2. Do you serve party foods that are high in fat and calories?	☐	☐	☐
3. Do you serve meals within fifteen minutes of the time you originally planned?	☐	☐	☐
4. Do you put serving dishes in the middle of your dining table for guests to help themselves from?	☐	☐	☐

	Yes	No	Unsure
5. Do your guests know at what time meals will be served?	☐	☐	☐
6. Do you always serve dessert at the end of meals?	☐	☐	☐
7. Do you offer guests low-calorie food and beverage choices if you know they have diabetes or are watching their weight?	☐	☐	☐
8. Do you urge guests to help themselves to second and third helpings of food?	☐	☐	☐
9. Do you allow guests to bring food or a dessert to share with your other guests?	☐	☐	☐
10. Do your guests tend to take naps, sit, or watch television after meals are over?	☐	☐	☐
11. Do your guests take walks or do some form of physical activity before and/or after meals?	☐	☐	☐

Results: Take a look at your responses. If you answered mostly "yes" to the odd-numbered questions (1, 3, 5, 7, 9, and 11) and "no" to the even-numbered questions (2, 4, 6, 8, and 10), your guests are well prepared to enjoy their day visiting you with minimal stress. They know what to expect and that they will be able to enjoy food and activities that are healthy for them.

If, however, you felt unsure answering some of the questions or responded with mostly "no" to the odd-numbered questions and "yes" to the even-numbered ones, some of your guests with diabetes may feel stressed trying to stick to their treatment plan when attending parties at your house. To help create a more supportive environment for them, consider talking with them before the holiday to learn what they find difficult versus helpful when attending special occasions at other people's houses. This will provide you with tips on how you can accommodate their unique health needs and ensure that they enjoy their visit to your place.

Q. What can I do to make holiday gatherings at my house special, while subtly providing support to someone who doesn't feel comfortable talking about his disease?

A. Holidays are an opportunity to gather with friends and loved ones, share special moments, and make lasting memories. While gatherings are meant to be fun, they can become stressful. Those hosting them can feel stressed when trying to anticipate the needs of all guests and worrying about making things go perfectly. This can result in trying to squeeze into their schedule last-minute preparations that require extra work or time. Those attending the event can become stressed when they aren't sure what to expect or if they know that the event will include foods they shouldn't eat.

Here are five simple, common courtesies to remember when planning for holiday gatherings to help ensure they are healthy and enjoyable for everyone attending. People with diabetes who may not feel comfortable talking about their condition are bound to appreciate your subtle efforts to put them at ease without making it look as if you've gone out of your way to give them special treatment.

Diabetiquette: Common Courtesies for Healthy, Stress-Free Holidays

Rule #1: Stay on Time
Be courteous and respectful of your guests' time by letting them know when they should arrive and when meals will be served. Once mealtimes are set, try to stay on time and serve meals within fifteen minutes of the established time. If someone is attending who has diabetes and takes either insulin or diabetes

pills, she will appreciate this gesture, as she could experience low blood glucose if the meal is delayed too long.

If some guests always arrive late, consider asking them to arrive a little earlier to build in a buffer zone so late arrivers will be there by the time your meal is ready. If the late arrivals are still not there, start serving the meal to the rest of your guests at the planned time. This way the guests who were on time don't miss out on eating the wonderful meal you've prepared for them, especially if some of the foods need to be served promptly so they don't dry out. When the late arrivals show up, kindly invite them to join in the meal and explain that you needed to start without them. Chances are, next time they won't be late!

Rule #2: Keep It Simple and Offer Choices

Sometimes holidays can seem to sneak up on us and throw our schedules into a tailspin of activities. Keeping up with family traditions can take a lot of work, time, and effort that can place extra stress on already busy calendars. However, holidays are meant to be joyous times that are calming to the soul and relaxing to the body.

If you and your family have expectations about what needs to happen during the holidays—what foods are made and decorations put up—it can sometimes feel like you're always rushing to get things done on time. If you find this to be true, try to create a holiday oasis for your guests—and you—by keeping your holiday gatherings simple. Determine which foods and activities absolutely need to be done versus those that are nice to have. If you're running short on time, cut back on those things that are nice to have but not essential to making the day a success. For example, instead of baking three or four different desserts,

---

How can I help? Remember the rules of diabetiquette when hosting parties: 1. Stay on time. 2. Keep it simple and offer choices. 3. Promote conversation, not food. 4. Include opportunities for people to be active before and after meals. 5. Relax and enjoy your special event.

decide to make only one or two and offer fresh fruit for health-conscious guests. When you have guests with diabetes, try to keep meals simple and well-balanced by offering choices from all the different food groups in the Food Guide Pyramid (see page 84). Don't forget to include sugar-free beverages like diet soft drinks, cocoa, or lemonade.

Remember, what's good for people with diabetes to eat is also good for everyone else. Other guests may be grateful when you serve low-calorie foods and offer more fresh fruits and vegetables.

Rule #3: Promote Conversation, Not Food

Do holiday meals revolve around food at your house? Do people look forward more to the food being served than seeing family and talking with each other? If they do, try to deemphasize the role of food and promote conversation and fellowship instead. For people with diabetes or who are trying to manage their weight, they will appreciate this effort and that you didn't tempt them to overeat.

There are three simple ways to encourage guests to focus more on talking and less about food. First, after people have been served their meal, place serving dishes with extra food on a table to the side of the dining table where everyone is sitting. Without everyone being overwhelmed by the amount of food available—tempting them to eat—they will focus more on each other and less on the food. This will encourage them to talk more about other subjects rather than just "pass the gravy and potatoes." Second, if you wish to offer people the opportunity to eat more, let them know they can. However, let them know they can help themselves or ask for what they would like passed to them. Try not to encourage people to "eat up" while passing around serving dishes. Let everyone decide for themselves how much to eat. Don't force food or drinks on people who say no, as it can encourage them to overeat when they are no longer hungry. Third, hold off serving desserts after large meals. Save dessert as a choice people can have a couple hours after a meal.

Rule #4: Include Opportunities for People to Be Active Before and After Meals

When your family gets together, are the adults just as active as the children? If not, encourage everyone to be more physically active on holidays. Besides being healthy for the heart and body, it helps relieve stress and creates opportunities for big and little kids alike to have fun together. If some guests usually settle down for naps or television after meals, encourage everyone to get up and take a short family walk around your neighborhood. Go to a park to get people moving and help them work off some of the calories they just ate at your wonderful meal. Consider playing with the children to create fond memories for them and you of holidays spent playing catch, learning to kick a soccer ball, or shooting baskets with relatives. If it's snowy outside, have a snowman or snow creature contest where everyone who can get outside helps to scoop up and mold snowmen. Elderly family members who aren't able to go outside can vote from a window or doorway to decide which is the most creative, the biggest, or the cutest. If it's sunny outside, wash and wax family cars together while a meal is grilling, or teach a child to fly a kite. If you're near a lake, take a boat ride together or go swimming.

Encouraging guests to be active will help guests with diabetes control their blood glucose level. At the same time, it gives guests who traveled long distances the chance to stretch their muscles instead of sitting all day.

Rule #5: Relax and Enjoy Your Special Event

When entertaining guests, don't get so busy caring for others that you forget to care for yourself and enjoy the holiday, too. Often, hosting a holiday gathering entails a lot of planning and work. During the course of the event, you may feel emotions ranging from happiness to frustration. You may worry whether guests like the food you prepare, especially those with diabetes. These are normal feelings and are to be expected. However, after the guests arrive and you get the meals served on time, ask for help if you need to finish up on things, like dishes. Then make time to talk with your guests and play games with the children. This way, you set a role model for everyone else that relaxing and enjoying each other's company is the most important thing to do on holidays—not washing dishes and cooking.

Q. This Thanksgiving and Christmas will be my husband's first holiday season having diabetes. He's not looking forward to it, as he can't eat many of his favorite foods anymore, for example, chutney, cranberry jelly, extra servings of stuffing, and cookies. He's not used to the idea of eating at scheduled times and watching his portion sizes. How can I help him enjoy the coming holiday season with our family?

A. Right now your husband is still adjusting and learning to cope with the idea of having a chronic illness. He's learning to accept the fact that his body isn't working like it used to anymore. His personal loss is forcing him to look at his habits and the changes he needs to make in his life to stay healthy. This can hurt and cause him to grieve. It's hard to change old habits—especially old habits he enjoyed, like munching on holiday cookies.

However, you can help him recognize his feelings and remember the purpose of the holidays, which is to make time in our lives to gather together with loved ones and friends to reflect on the past, enjoy the present, and refresh our souls to look with hope toward the future. You can help him identify foods that he enjoys that are healthy for him to eat (such as turkey, mashed potatoes, a small portion of stuffing, and sweet potatoes) so he understands that he doesn't have to give up all of his favorite foods. Offer to find recipes that adapt some of his favorite high-calorie foods to make them fit his new way of eating. This way he may see that with a little tweaking of fat and sugar in a recipe, he can still enjoy some of his favorite foods if he eats them in moderation at his meals.

For recipe ideas, explore some of the cookbooks listed at the end of this book (see pages 257–258). You can find them at your local bookstore and possibly at your local library.

Q. My family has many holiday traditions that center around food and sitting. However, I'd like to start some new traditions that are healthy and simple to do. How can I start?

A. While there are many older traditions that are beautiful and full of meaning (e.g., religious or cultural customs and family activities), new traditions can gain similar meaning when they can be enjoyed by young and old alike. The idea of creating new traditions shouldn't seem scary, or mean that you're replacing (giving up) all of your previous traditions. Instead, remember that traditions are the beliefs, customs, information, and activities that you wish to pass down to the generation that comes after you. They can consist of things both large and small. It can be as simple as giving everyone hugs as they enter and leave your home or planning a family recreational activity. If you reflect back on your youth, often the fondest memories are the simple acts of kindness and time spent with family and friends as people worked on activities together. As your family looks to make new traditions, consider what you want children to remember and cherish as memories. Be creative.

Here are some ideas that may be fun to do.

- *Playing cards.* Help young children read numbers and learn arithmetic by teaching them how to play your family's favorite card games. This can provide years of inexpensive family enjoyment as you meet for holiday gatherings.

- *Walking.* Enjoy the outside air by getting out and walking together. Keep young children entertained and see the world through their eyes for a few minutes playing a game of "find-it." Make a list of things for children to find as you're walking and see who's the first person to spot all the items. For example, see who can find the first red car, the first garage door that has a window on it, the first fire hydrant, the first cracked sidewalk, or the first butterfly.

- *Volunteering.* On holidays, if you want to help brighten someone else's day, consider volunteering to help someone less fortunate. There's nothing that lifts the spirit more than knowing you helped someone. Consider volunteering as a family to feed the homeless, sing carols at a local hospital, visit old friends and neighbors at nursing homes, repaint a house for someone elderly, or bring a special meal to someone who is housebound or ill.

- *Exercising.* Consider building exercise into the family gathering. Play tennis, golf, table tennis, or Frisbee, go sledding, ride horses, ski, play basketball, or swim together. If you live near a park or have a large back yard, teach children how to play favorite family games like croquet, bocce ball, badminton, or horseshoes, which they can play against relatives of all ages.

- *Sharing talents.* Have family singalongs around a bonfire or around a piano where you can have family members teach each other songs and appreciate each other's talents. Have children perform puppet skits, or adults lead in storytelling.

- *Hunting for treasure.* Have a scavenger or Easter egg hunt by having older family members hide clues or items inside or outside the house and having the rest of the family hunt to see

> *How can I help?*
> Promote family traditions that revolve around the inner meaning of holidays and spending time with friends and family rather than focusing solely around food.

who can find a family treasure first. Search individually or in teams, matching relatives and friends of different ages.

Q. Do I have to give up eating all of my favorite holiday foods just because my spouse has diabetes? I don't have diabetes or need to watch out for fat in my diet.

A. You're right. You do not have diabetes and do not need to change how you eat. However, the fact is that someone close to you has an illness where she does need to watch what she eats. Whether you deny the fact or not, you will play a positive or negative role in supporting her efforts to successfully cope with diabetes. If you ignore her needs and require that she eat the foods you like, it makes it hard for her to make the choices she needs to make to stay healthy. However, if you decide to work with her to control her diabetes, together you will see that you don't have to give up all your favorite foods. Many holiday foods can be prepared in lower-fat ways by just tweaking an ingredient or two. You can also decide to cook fewer of the holiday foods so that there are fewer leftovers around to tempt her to eat foods that are inappropriate for her diet. It's your decision how supportive you will be.

Q. My parents' fortieth wedding anniversary is next month, and I'm trying to plan a party for them. But I'm not sure what to serve because my mom has diabetes and shouldn't eat sweets. What should I do? Should I make her a cake?

A. If you're not sure what to do for your parents and what to serve at a family gathering, the answer is simple: Ask them what they would like. Celebrating anniversaries is a way friends and family can honor a couple's achievements in life. They are occasions that bring people together who may not have seen each other for many years. They are a time of reminiscing, reflecting, and sharing friendship. Find out what would be most meaningful to them.

Determine if they would prefer a special meal with their immediate family, eating out at a favorite restaurant so no one has to cook or clean up a meal, or having a reception at a local center that encourages socializing among extended family and friends. For the meal, follow the guidelines discussed earlier in this section and you'll be set to celebrate! As for sweets, depending upon your mother's diabetes control, she may say that a small cake is fine. If this is the case, make or purchase a simple decorated layer cake that is lightly frosted. By planning ahead, your mother can have a small middle piece of cake (not a corner piece with oodles of frosting) with her meal. Or your mother may decide that she would like to have a different dessert instead of a traditional cake (e.g., having your own ice cream sundaes with light vanilla ice cream and a variety of toppings, including fresh fruit).

How can I help?   *If you celebrate anniversaries, weddings, and birthdays with cake, avoid ordering too large a cake. If you do, send the leftovers home with friends and family who don't have diabetes and can easily eat it up, instead of with those who may end up throwing it out.*

Q. My daughter is getting married in a couple of months, and her fiancé has diabetes. We're trying to plan a reception, dinner, and dance for them. What should we keep in mind while we're planning the event?

A. Weddings are exciting occasions. Depending upon how elaborate the festivities will be, wedding gatherings can last from a few hours with a simple ceremony and reception to an entire weekend that includes a rehearsal dinner, ceremony, family events, and opening gifts. In addition to the usual wedding plans for decorations, invitations, and apparel, here are some tips to keep in mind to help someone getting married keep their diabetes under control.

Pre-Wedding Checklist

- ☐ Try to coordinate the times of all meals to coincide with the usual times when the person with diabetes eats.
- ☐ Remember to include noncaloric beverages for guests (e.g., coffee, tea, sugar-free fruit drinks or soft drinks).
- ☐ When preparing the wedding meal, remember to include food from each of the six food groups of the food pyramid.
- ☐ When preparing the wedding meal, offer foods that are baked, broiled, grilled, or steamed instead of foods that are fried or have cream sauces.
- ☐ Include a light or reduced-fat salad dressing option if serving salad—serve dressings on the side.
- ☐ Consider offering guests healthy foods as a late night snack at dances where people will be active (e.g., popcorn, pretzels, raw vegetables, or leftover fresh fruit if served at the dinner).

Wedding Day Checklist to Help Keep Glucose Levels Under Control

Enlist the assistance of the best man, maid of honor, or personal attendant to:

☐ ensure that the person with diabetes gets plenty of sleep the night before the wedding.

☐ ensure that the person with diabetes does not skip meals or forget to eat in their excitement at getting married.

☐ double-check that the person's diabetes supplies (meter, pills, or insulin and syringe) are located in an easily accessible place before and after the wedding and reception.

☐ remind the person with diabetes to take their insulin or medication before the wedding meal, if needed.

☐ carry some form of fast-acting glucose (e.g., glucose tabs) with them in their pocket or purse in case the person with diabetes needs to quickly treat hypoglycemia symptoms.

☐ caution the person against drinking alcohol (during a reception) on an empty stomach, which could put them at risk for hypoglycemia.

☐ make sure that the person with diabetes gets to the dinner on time (no kidnapping the bride or groom for a few minutes of fun that would delay eating dinner on time).

☐ make sure the person with diabetes packs a form of fast-acting glucose in his luggage in case he needs to treat hypoglycemia on the wedding night. It's better to be safe and ready to treat than have to hunt for something to use as a treatment late at night or in the morning.

Q. My husband, who has diabetes, and I are hoping to take a vacation this summer to visit friends in another state. We're afraid his diabetes will get out of control when eating away from home so much. What should we keep in mind as we plan our trip?

A. Whether traveling for a day or a week, by planning ahead you can see the sights, eat out, and keep your husband's diabetes under control. It's possible to do. Here's how.

After you decide on your destination, you'll need to also decide how you're going to get there. If you travel by car, plan to stop for meals and snacks at the times he usually eats. Keep his usual schedule going. Carry a small cooler with you in the car to keep a handy supply of beverages, fresh fruit, vegetables, and sandwich fixings in case you are unable to find a restaurant or experience traffic delays. Instead of eating at fast food restaurants, which may offer few selections, try eating at sandwich shops and restaurants where you can select from a variety of menu options to fit his dietary needs. Don't leave any insulin or blood glucose monitoring equipment in a car, where it could be exposed to very hot or very cold temperatures—this can be harmful to his diabetes supplies.

If you decide to travel by plane, find out if meals will be served on the plane or not. Many airlines offer special meals for people with diabetes if you request them at the time you purchase your tickets. They also usually stock sugar-free soft drinks and juice as beverages that are available if you ask for them. In case of plane delays or layovers, plan to carry a few healthy snacks with you in your purse or carry-on baggage to tide you and your husband over until you can eat your meal. Also, have your husband always carry his diabetes supplies, insulin, and medication with him on the plane so they arrive with him at your destination (in case the airlines accidentally lose his luggage).

Last but not least, don't forget to have your husband carry identification with him that indicates he has diabetes. If he doesn't wear a medical alert ID, he should at least carry something in his wallet along with the emergency phone numbers for his doctor and insurance company. He may wish to carry an extra prescription for insulin, medications, and supplies with him in case he runs out and needs to purchase them in a different state. If he's traveling overseas, he may wish to carry a brief medical record and a signed statement from his physician saying that he has diabetes and uses medication. As the Boy Scouts say, always be prepared!

How can I help? When dining out at unfamiliar restaurants, observe the size and type of meals other diners are eating. Ask how the food is prepared and if you can substitute lower-fat food items like fruit, salad, or soup for fried potatoes. If meals are large, consider splitting a meal with your friend with diabetes.In most cases, restaurants are happy to oblige special requests if you take the time to ask.

Q. My grandson with diabetes is coming to visit me without his parents for a week after he finishes elementary school this spring. Is there anything I should keep in mind as I prepare to have him stay with me?

A. Having grandchildren visit can be exciting for both grandparents and grandchildren. When a child has diabetes, it's important that grandparents try their best to keep the child's meal and activity schedule as close as possible to his usual routine at home. Keeping him on a consistent schedule will help him adjust more quickly to being in a new environment.

While spoiling grandchildren is something grandparents love to do, it's best to find ways to do so that don't involve food. For example, it's common in our society to treat children to candy and sweets. If you're out shopping with your grandson, don't splurge and buy him a lollipop or ice cream cone. While it's an easy thing to do, it can affect his blood glucose level if it does not fit into his diet. If this happens, he may not feel well. Instead, ask his parents for nonfood ways you can spoil him; for example, give him oodles of attention and listen to him tell you stories, buy him a new toy or outfit, read books with him, play games, or take him to the video arcade, zoo, or a sports game.

Before he visits, talk with his parents to learn how they manage his diabetes and what food he normally eats. Here are questions to help you prepare to care for him.

Safety Checklist for Stayovers or Babysitting

☐ At what times does he normally eat?

☐ What does he normally eat for meals and snacks?

☐ Are there foods that he usually doesn't eat?

☐ Can he care for his own diabetes, or does he need help checking his blood glucose level or injecting insulin?

☐ What symptoms does he get when his blood glucose level is low (hypoglycemia)?

☐ How much insulin does he take and when?

☐ How should you treat hypoglycemia, should he have it?

☐ At what point during a hypoglycemia episode should you call his parents or seek emergency care?

☐ What symptoms does he get when his blood glucose level is high (hyperglycemia)?

☐ How does his blood glucose meter work?

☐ When should he test his blood glucose level?

☐ Are there precautions you should take before letting him go out to play?

☐ Will his parents sign a waiver slip authorizing you to have him medically treated in case of an emergency if you're unable to reach them? Obtain pertinent health insurance information.

☐ Obtain the phone number of his health care provider in case of an illness or emergency.

☐ Have parents create a list of nonfood ways grandparents can spoil their grandchild.

How can I help?
Remember to avoid having children with diabetes play strenuously right before meals, as it puts them at risk for hypoglycemia.

Q. I'm on a church committee that's planning a weekend workshop for seniors, of whom many attending have diabetes. What should I keep in mind as we plan the meals?

A. When planning meals and snacks for conferences, you will want to offer foods that are healthy for everyone. Besides being healthy, serving lower-fat meals will also help prevent participants from feeling tired after eating. This is because high-fat meals can give people a feeling of fullness and satiety that can make them feel sluggish. Here are some tips to consider when planning a conference or workshop.

Encourage Stretching Activities

- During session breaks, encourage people to walk around and stretch their legs by letting them know where they can go for a quick walk.

- Select conference sites near shopping areas or parks—this can motivate people to walk around to stretch and thus help increase their attention span during the sessions.

- Select conference hotels that offer exercise equipment rooms, pools, or access to other activities for guests to use before and after meeting sessions.

Serve Healthy Meals

- Include something from each different food group at each meal, using the Food Guide Pyramid as your guide

- Serve potatoes, pasta, rice, and vegetables without heavy cream sauces.

- Offer salads made with sugar-free gelatin or fresh vegetables with low-calorie dressing.

- Offer sugar-free beverages.

- If serving dessert, consider something light like a fruit cup or small dish of frozen yogurt.

- Serve sauces, gravies, and condiments on the side so that participants can decide for themselves how much they wish to use.

Q. I'm hoping to invite a new neighbor over to join my card club. I heard she has diabetes. What kind of snacks can I serve that she can eat?

A. If the purpose of your card club is to play cards and visit, try not to let food become a focal point of your gathering. Depending upon what time your club meets, you may decide that food is not necessary. Often people are satisfied with flavorful beverages to sip on while they play. If, however, you decide food must be part of your gathering, then what to serve will depend on when you're meeting. If you're planning on gathering near a mealtime, you may want to serve a mini-meal before or after you play cards. If you're meeting between meals, offer beverages and light snacks (see the list below) that are low in calories. Don't push food on your guests, in case someone doesn't want to snack between meals. Let her graciously decline a snack if she wants to. Also, don't keep snacks on the table as you play. Besides taking up valuable space on the card table, they create an attractive temptation for someone to munch on, which can affect her blood glucose control and efforts to manage her weight.

Light Snack Ideas

- baked tortilla chips with salsa
- low-fat pretzels
- flavored rice crackers/cakes
- biscotti and hot or chilled coffee
- fresh vegetables: green beans, carrots, celery, broccoli florets, jicama or rutabaga strips, cauliflower, low-fat dip
- shortbread and flavored tea
- popcorn sprinkled with parmesan cheese
- icy-cold sugar-free lemonade
- baked bagel chips and hummus
- fresh fruit cups with lemon yogurt (nonfat) topping
- low-fat chocolate mousse with a pirouette cookie
- low-fat quick dessert breads

CHAPTER 6

Creating Positive Work Environments

During the course of one's life, it's not uncommon to spend many hours—sometimes countless hours—working with other people, sometimes the same people for months or years. It may be with people you work with at your job, at church, or at volunteer programs. While working together, friendships can develop between people that forge strong bonds, bonds sometimes almost as strong as those in a family. These bonds create what can be called "work families." Within a work family, people know when someone's having a good day or feeling frustrated. In times of stress or trouble, people console and support each other, while at other times they celebrate each other's joys and achievements. You may think you know each other pretty well, but you'll still be amazed sometimes that you don't know everything.

If diabetes affects someone you work with who is part of your work family, the news may affect you a little or a lot, depending on how close you are to that person. You may be curious about how and when he got diabetes. You may wonder how he treats it, if he's doing okay, or even if he will be able to keep doing his job. As you learn more about diabetes and how it's treated, you may become concerned with how he and his family are adjusting and coping with the disease. You may think about how you'd react to being diagnosed with diabetes and maybe even ponder the meaning of life for a few minutes. Because you're reading this book, you are definitely interested in knowing if there's some way you can help. The answer is, yes, you can.

Whether you are a coworker or manager, you can help support and encourage a person at work who has diabetes to take good care of himself. You can help create a work environment that supports healthy lifestyle habits and is diabetes-friendly. This chapter will show you ways to do this. It will help you assess your workplace and organizational culture to identify any barriers that could create diabetes self-care challenges. The chapter will review how diabetes is legally a disability and how current laws prevent discrimination in the workplace. Last but not least, the chapter will help you establish an action plan should someone with diabetes become hypoglycemic at work.

Q. Growing up in the late 1950s, I remember my brother, who has diabetes, being told by our doctor not to plan on going to college or having a career, as his health wouldn't allow it. But he went on to earn several college degrees and just retired, a successful businessman. Is it common now for people with diabetes to have careers?

A. It's true that in the past, people with diabetes were sometimes told by their doctor that diabetes would affect their ability to have a career and/or a family. This was based on how diabetes was treated in the early 1900s and how little was known at the time about the quality of life someone could lead while treated with insulin. As new types of insulin, medications, and research became available, the barriers that existed that caused people to fear that those with diabetes wouldn't live long or have a high quality of life were removed.

Today, there are few restrictions limiting people with diabetes from achieving their dream of going to college, having careers, and raising families. Those like your brother who have lived with diabetes for over fifty years show the world that their disease doesn't have to stop them from enjoying life. They looked beyond their disease to identify what they wanted to achieve in life and went after it.

Q. I've been Jerry's manager for five years and just learned he's had diabetes most of his life. I never had a clue because he had never said a word about it. Isn't there a law somewhere that requires people to report this kind of thing when they are hired?

A. Actually, according to the Americans with Disabilities Act, people with diabetes are not required by law to report when they apply for a job that they have a chronic disease. This law was created to prevent people with disabilities—like diabetes—from being discriminated against or not considered for employment based on having a medical condition. While employers are allowed to *ask* job applicants to identify themselves as having a disability, they cannot *require* people to report it.

If a person with diabetes receives and accepts a job offer, he only needs to disclose his condition if he's required to complete a medical exam as part of being hired, like everyone else the employer hires.

Having diabetes should not limit someone from being hired for any job they are qualified for and able to do. Employers can actually benefit from hiring talented people with diabetes, as it complies with federal affirmative action laws.

Q. Why do some people hide the fact that they have diabetes?

A. While many people with diabetes do share with managers and coworkers the fact that they have it, some don't, for a variety of personal reasons. First, their decision may be influenced by past experiences they've had in telling other people. If the news in the past wasn't received well, it could make them leery to tell others for fear of being treated differently. Second, their decision not to tell may be based on their personality type and cultural beliefs. They may feel that their disease is a private matter, to be shared only on a need-to-know basis. Third, they may not openly talk about their disease if they haven't yet come to terms with the fact that they have a chronic illness.

If you have never had a chronic illness or disability, it may be hard for you to understand the many feelings a person with diabetes can experience. You may think, "What's the big deal about telling someone you have diabetes?" To help you gain a glimpse of what concerns they may have, try putting yourself in their shoes for a few minutes. Try the experiment below.

To Tell or Not to Tell—Which Would I Do?

Imagine this morning you were relaxing in your living room reading a newspaper. Suddenly your phone rang. You jumped up and rushed to the kitchen to answer it. Unfortunately, in your haste, you accidentally stepped on a toy truck (metal, of course) that your son forgot to put away last night. Ouch!

While the toy survived the accident, your foot wasn't as lucky. Besides missing the phone call, your foot is now bruised and there's a cut on the side of your big toe that needs bandaging.

As you get ready for work, you discover you can't wear your usual work shoes, because they hurt your sore foot and toe. Consequently, you end up wearing open-toed sandals to work, as they are the only pair of shoes you can tolerate walking in.

As your read the following questions, check the box next to the response that best describes what would happen if you limped into work wearing sandals.

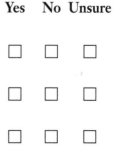

	Yes	No	Unsure
1. Will others at work notice you have a sore foot if you don't tell them?	☐	☐	☐
2. Does anyone at work need to know you have a sore foot?	☐	☐	☐
3. Will people treat you differently because you have a sore foot?	☐	☐	☐

	Yes	No	Unsure
4. Does having a sore foot make you less qualified or able to do your job?	☐	☐	☐
5. Is it okay for you to wear sandals at work until your foot is better?	☐	☐	☐

> *Results:* Depending on what kind of job you pictured yourself doing, it's possible to answer the questions in a number of different ways. If you sit at a desk all day in a casual work environment, you probably answered "no" to most of the questions. Having a sore foot wouldn't affect how well you did your job or be noticed by anyone when your feet are under your desk. However, if you do a job where you either stand or walk a lot, you may have answered "unsure" or "yes" to some of the questions. You may have received some curious stares from coworkers or been questioned as to why you were limping. This would have forced you to decide whether you wanted to tell the truth (you stepped on a toy) or not. Other than some teasing, telling your friends and coworkers about your accident probably wouldn't affect your ability to do your job. However, if wearing closed-toe shoes was a requirement in your work area for safety or dress code reasons, your supervisor may have told you to change your shoes or reassigned your duties for the day.

Now instead of having a sore toe, imagine that you have a serious medical condition like HIV infection, epilepsy, or cancer. Ask yourself the same questions, inserting the disease name where the blanks are. See if you answer the questions as quickly or in the same way as you did before.

	Yes	No	Unsure
1. Will others at work notice you have _____ if you don't tell them?	☐	☐	☐
2. Does anyone at work need to know you have _____?	☐	☐	☐

	Yes	No	Unsure
3. Will people treat you differently because you have _____?	☐	☐	☐
4. Does having _____ make you less qualified or able to do your job?	☐	☐	☐
5. Can you adjust your work area to help you cope with having _____?	☐	☐	☐

Results: If you found yourself wanting to answer, "Well, it would depend on . . . " or "It's none of their business" or some as "yes" or "unsure," you are now relating to the dilemma people with diabetes have when trying to decide whether to tell people around them about their health problem. To tell or not to tell isn't always an easy (clear-cut or black-and-white) decision to make. It's a personal decision that needs to be made on a case-to-case basis, depending on the situation one is in.

Those who have learned to cope with their diabetes may find it easier to talk to others and be open about their disease. This doesn't mean that they run up to everyone they meet announcing, "Hi, I'm Sharon and I have diabetes." It just means that if having diabetes comes up in a conversation, they feel comfortable talking about it. They don't hide the fact that they have it. A *Diabetes Forecast* magazine readers' survey reported that three out of four people with diabetes want to let people know they have diabetes, because they're proud of the hard work they do to control it. Also, 88 percent believe it's good to tell people about their diabetes so that others learn more about the disease. To them, diabetes is just something they have and need to manage daily.

How can I help? Get to know the people you work with—know your work family! Learn who they are, appreciate each other's strengths and differences, and respect each other's right to have feelings that may be different from your own.

In contrast, those who haven't accepted or learned to cope with the fact that they have a chronic illness (which can take months or years to do) may not be as open to talking about it. Their coping method may be to act as normal as possible while they come to grips with the fact that their body isn't acting normally anymore. They may hide their diabetes from their coworkers and even their family for fear of what people will think and how they might be treated if they knew.

Q. I work with Jeff, who has diabetes. He doesn't look sick or act disabled. In fact, he plays on our company softball team and is our best player. I don't understand why he is considered disabled. Can you explain this?

A. The terms "normal" and "disabled" are words we use to label people as we try to describe differences amongst each other. While those with diabetes look and act normal on the outside, internally their bodies don't act in a normal fashion, as they have a problem regulating their blood glucose level.

How disabilities are defined and assessed varies slightly between research studies and agencies. One definition defines disabilities in relation to impairments. For example, a glucose impairment causes a person's blood glucose level to be either above or below normal—out of control. When this occurs, it causes symptoms that affect how well the body functions or acts (for example, seeing, thinking, or walking). When the blood glucose level remains poorly controlled over long periods of time, impairments can become permanent and restrict one's ability to perform certain activities. When this happens, it's called a disability.

Does this sound complicated? It's not when you consider an example. Imagine that someone with diabetes was a professional baseball player. If he became hypoglycemic during a game, it would temporarily affect his ability to hit or catch a ball. After the low is treated, however, his symptoms would subside and he'd feel back to "normal"—ready to return to the game. However, if the baseball player didn't care for his diabetes, over time he could develop complications from his disease. Were his vision to become permanently blurry, he could no longer see a baseball being pitched to him, and he wouldn't be able to play professionally anymore. At this point, his diabetes would turn from being an impairment that didn't affect his ability to play ball to a disability restricting him from doing his previously normal activities.

According to the Americans with Disabilities Act, people are legally considered disabled in one of three ways:

1. They have a physical or mental impairment that limits to a large extent one or more major life activity, for example, caring for oneself, walking, seeing, hearing, speaking, breathing, and working. Physical and mental impairments include conditions like visual, speech or hearing impairments, diabetes, heart disease, cancer, AIDS, mental retardation, or drug addiction.

2. They have a record of ever having had a physical or mental impairment.

3. Others view them as having an impairment (even though they may not feel disabled).

Diabetes is a physical impairment that can affect one's ability to do normal activities of daily living if it's not treated. However, to legally prove someone is disabled, one must still be substantially limited in a major life activity after receiving medication or treatment for a condition.

Q. How many people with diabetes are disabled?

A. Technically, everyone with diabetes can be considered disabled (per the legal definition above), because they all have a glucose impairment. However, legally not all fit the definition after taking medication as not everyone with diabetes is limited in performing physical activities.

In 1994, the Centers for Disease Control reported that half of all people with diabetes viewed themselves as having activity limitations to some degree. Activity limitations were defined as not being able to perform daily activities such as going to work or school, doing housekeeping, or caring for oneself.

As people with diabetes got older, the number reporting physical disabilities increased. Only 10 percent of people with type 1 diabetes under the age of 44 report having physical limitations. However, this rate increases to almost 50 percent after age 45. In contrast, 45 percent of people with type 2 diabetes between the ages of 18 and 44 report having physical limitations, and the rate increases to above 55 percent after age 45. Disabilities are also more commonly seen in those who have developed diabetes complications.

As people become physically disabled, the effects of their condition result in higher rates of unemployment, more absenteeism (lost days from work), higher use of health care services, and a perceived decrease in one's quality of life.

Q. Does having diabetes really make it hard for someone to get or hold a job?

A. It's unfortunate, but true. People have been denied jobs and employment opportunities based upon the single fact that they had diabetes. Because some work policies allow no exceptions, some have lost their jobs regardless of how well their diabetes was controlled or their ability to do a job.

In Arizona and North Carolina, two school bus drivers battled against diabetes discrimination in their states and won. Both were drivers with longstanding, accident-free driving records who also happened to have diabetes. To achieve the best diabetes control they could, both needed to change their diabetes treatment plan to include insulin. However, once their states' motor vehicle departments learned they were using insulin, their licenses to drive buses were taken away, which resulted in them both losing their jobs. To their dismay, each state had blanket policies that automatically banned people using insulin to treat diabetes from driving buses.

In 1998, the U.S. Department of Justice intervened and declared that the state policies were inconsistent with the federal

Americans with Disabilities Act. The policies were discriminatory, as they were based upon an old belief that people who take insulin to treat diabetes were unsafe drivers! The policies failed to consider someone's driving skills, their ability to do their job, or how well their diabetes was controlled. Consequently, the two cases were settled and resulted in both states revising their driver policies to reflect the fact that diabetes is a treatable disease. Diabetes doesn't have to be a barrier to someone being an effective worker.

Another example of job discrimination involved airplane pilots. Prior to 1996, the Federal Aviation Administration (FAA) banned people with insulin-treated diabetes from piloting planes.

For thirty-seven years, its policy allowed people to fly only if they were able to treat their diabetes without insulin (with medications, diet, and exercise). However, if they needed to use insulin, their wings were stripped from them, which resulted in pilots losing their jobs. The policy automatically prohibited people with type 1 diabetes from flying. However, it also resulted in many pilots with type 2 diabetes having poor glucose control, as they delayed starting insulin therapy so they could hang onto their jobs. In 1996, the FAA revised its policy. It now allows people with insulin-treated diabetes to apply for individual consideration to pilot aircraft based on their ability to fly, their medical history, and blood glucose monitoring records that prove they have good diabetes control.

It's unfortunate, but because some employers have hung onto old fears and beliefs that people with diabetes are too big a risk to employ, people with diabetes have had to sometimes struggle to get employment policies updated to reflect new diabetes treatment plans to overcome this prejudice. Fortunately, with the help of the Americans with Disabilities Act, employment opportunities for people with diabetes have improved. Today, people with diabetes hold jobs ranging from farmers, lawyers, government leaders, health care providers, truck drivers, and professional athletes to musicians, teachers, office employees, and rescue personnel.

Savvy employers are also discovering a secret—people with diabetes can make exceptional employees because they often have the very traits employers look for in employees. Because they're forced to cope with a chronic disease, people with diabetes often take better care of their health than people without diabetes by eating healthy diets, exercising regularly, and managing their weight and stress levels. Managing their blood glucose levels requires self-discipline, being able to stay on schedule, and problem-solving skills. You couldn't ask for better qualities in employees!

> *How can I help?*
> Don't be afraid to hire someone with diabetes if he is qualified and able to do the job. Diabetes doesn't have to be a barrier to enjoying life and being a good employee.

Q. How, exactly, does the Americans with Disabilities Act protect people with diabetes against discrimination at work?

A. The Americans with Disabilities Act is a federal civil rights law that protects against discrimination and unfair treatment in the same way civil rights laws protect people from discrimination on the basis of their race, age, color, sex, and religion. Its goal is to protect against discrimination with regard to hiring, firing, advancement, training, tenure, leave, compensation, and other employment-related activities. However, the act fails to protect everyone with diabetes.

Originally passed in 1990 (and revised a few times since), the Americans with Disabilities Act applies to the following employers: all federal, state, and local governments, employment agencies, labor unions, transportation, telecommunications, and any company that has at least fifteen employees. Some cities and states have additional antidiscrimination laws that go beyond the scope of the federal act.

For the act to work, employers first need to know that an employee has a disability. If the person with diabetes hasn't told anyone that she has diabetes, then she can't possibly be discriminated against on the basis of her disease. The act protects her only when the employer knows and regards her as disabled, and she establishes she is protected by the law because of physical limitations.

Once an employer knows an applicant has diabetes and is protected by the act, he is required to provide reasonable accommodation so she is able to do her job. Reasonable accommodation simply means that either the job duties, work area, or work schedule can be adjusted to help her perform her job, if needed. This could consist of providing a special computer keyboard so she has an easier time typing or doing data entry, or allowing either consistent or flexible break times. However, if what it would take to accommodate an employee is either unreasonable or would cause undue hardship on the operation of a company (for instance, cost too much or be unrealistic), an employer doesn't have to hire that person. In 1999, the Supreme Court ruled that if a person is not limited by their diabetes after being treated with medications and/or prescriptive devices and doesn't establish with their employer they are covered under a disability act or antidiscriminatory law, an employer can legally deny hiring and even fire someone because of their disease.

Q. Do the discrimination laws protect people outside the workforce?

A. Yes. The Americans with Disabilities Act can protect family, roommates, and friends of those with diabetes from unfair treatment based on their relationship with the person with diabetes. It also protects the rights of people with diabetes who don't work but are treated differently because they have a disease, for example, students and retired individuals.

Discrimination can happen at any age level and in places besides the work setting. It can happen to children in school and to older adults in retirement. In 1998, the Equal Employment Opportunities Commission reported that between 1992 and 1997, almost 3,300 complaints alleging diabetes discrimination had been filed.

One complaint that was filed was against day care centers on behalf of infants and toddlers with diabetes. In 1996 and 1997, the U.S. Department of Justice ruled that KinderCare and La Petite Academy, two national day care providers, had broken the Americans with Disabilities Act when they didn't allow children with diabetes to enroll in their centers. The centers didn't want to take children who needed to do daily blood glucose (finger-stick) tests. As a result, day care centers around the country were reminded to treat children fairly. They needed to help monitor children's blood glucose levels (if requested by parents), observe their special dietary needs, and alert parents if blood glucose levels fell outside agreed-upon ranges.

> **How can I help?**
> Remember, you're a work family. Within families, take the time to get to know each other and how to best support each other so everyone can succeed.

Q. As a manager, I don't think I've discriminated against any of my employees. However, I'm not sure. Is there a way to assess if I have accidentally done so?

A. When discrimination happens, most of the time it's unintentional. Usually people don't go around thinking, "Today I'm going to pick on someone who's disabled or has diabetes." That's not considered acceptable behavior in our society. However, it can happen accidentally.

To discriminate against someone, by definition, means that you treat someone differently from everyone else on the basis of things other than his ability to do a job on merit. When it happens, it's often a decision based on factors outside one's control (e.g., age, race, color of skin, or gender). To help you identify your risk for discriminating against someone with diabetes, take the following quiz.

> **How can I help?**
> To remain fair and be respected by employees, always pick the best person for the job based on skills and merit.

How Fair Am I?

Directions: Answer the following questions by checking the response that most closely matches how you would react in the following situations.

1. You are a manager and need someone to attend a dinner meeting in your absence. You'd like to ask Whitney to attend, but debate asking her because she has diabetes and always eats dinner at a certain time. You decide to:

   A. Ask Matt because he's single and probably has a more flexible schedule.

   B. Ask Carrie because she likes to eat fried fish, which is what they are serving at the dinner.

   C. Ask Whitney and let her decide if she can attend or not in your place.

2. You need to promote a new head secretary for your department. Your first thought is to promote Wendy, but then you remember she has diabetes and doesn't like to work late (overtime). You decide to offer the job to:

   A. Todd because he's pretty good using computers and doesn't mind working late.

   B. Katie because she's worked longest in the department and is a peach of a person.

   C. Wendy because she's the most qualified candidate.

3. You're chosen to put together a task force to decide which food service company will get the contract to run the cafeteria at work for the next three years. You need someone on the task force who has accounting experience and are considering whether to ask Bruce or Elise. You decide to:

   A. Pick Elise because she's always munching on snack foods and women are better at food stuff.

   B. Pick Bruce because he has diabetes and plays on your softball team at work.

C. Ask them both and see who has a stronger interest in joining.

4. You're a talent scout and need to hire one more person to join a traveling theater group performing the musical *Grease!* You've narrowed the field down to three candidates. You hire Dick for the following reason:

A. He seems the healthiest, so he wouldn't need much for medical benefits.

B. He looks the most like John Travolta—tall, dark-haired, and white.

C. He dances the jitterbug and lindy the best.

5. You're planning a slumber party for your daughter's eighth birthday. She wants to invite nine friends, but you have set a limit of eight. You advise her to:

A. Invite only the girls on her list, which would automatically eliminate her best friend, Tom.

B. Not invite Emily because you don't want to take the risk that she could have an insulin reaction while she's at your house.

C. List her closest (best) eight friends and invite them first, saving the ninth person as an alternate if someone can't attend.

Results

If you answered C for all of the questions—congratulations! By picking a person based upon personal merit, skills, or abilities, you selected the fairest options for each situation.

If you answered A or B for some of the questions, you may occasionally treat people unfairly. Be careful when making decisions to not let personal traits sway you; for instance, the color of someone's hair or skin, their weight or appearance, religion, marital status, or any medical condition. Make your decision on the basis of who's most deserving. Once you make your pick, it's up to him to decide if he can or can't accept your proposal.

Q. As a manager, do I need to give people with diabetes special treatment?

A. People with diabetes usually don't need or request special treatment—they just want to be treated fairly. Good managers who care for their employees know that emotionally and physically healthy employees are more productive and satisfied in their jobs than those who are frustrated, stressed, feeling unappreciated, or coping with physical ailments. Good managers take time to know their employees and learn what's important to them. They try to create a work environment where all employees can succeed and contribute to the success of their organization. Thus, they turn their work family into a high-performance work team.

As a manager, it's your job to know who makes up your work family and how to empower them to be successful. If you have someone working for you with diabetes, you need to take the time to understand how she treats her disease. If you don't take the time, you could contribute (unintentionally) to creating barriers for her that make it hard for her to manage her diabetes well.

For example, imagine that you have an important project deadline, which includes writing a report by the end of the day. You're not done yet, so you decide to call an employee or fellow coworker to request that she promptly supply you with information or help you write part of the report. When you call her, do you consider what project she is working on, or do you expect her to drop what she's doing and help you immediately? Do you know what kind of impact your request has on the rest of her day and completing her own work? Do you know if the deadline you just gave her is realistic, or whether it will increase her stress level—while yours goes down? Do you expect her to skip or delay her lunch or break to meet your deadline?

High-functioning work families make conscious efforts to respect each other's time and health. As a manager, you need to help your employees establish realistic goals for what can be accomplished within normal work hours that include time for breaks and lunch. Not recognizing the need for breaks can contribute to a stressful environment for both you and those around you. For those with diabetes who use insulin or diabetes pills, skipping or delaying lunch could cause them to become hypoglycemic—the last thing anyone would want to happen.

This doesn't mean that you can't ask someone to work overtime or meet tight deadlines. It just means you can't forget the fact that, unlike you, she has a disease that requires her to maintain a meal schedule. So the next time deadlines are tight, an easy solution would be to give her a couple of options on how she could help. One option may be to let her eat her lunch at her desk while she works so she doesn't need to delay her medical treatment and lunch. Another option would be to let her take a short lunch break, followed by a stretch break later in the day after the deadline is met. A third option would be to model the importance of lunch breaks and take a mini one together. This way you both can relax for a few minutes, catch your breath, and work more effectively during the afternoon to meet your deadline. By taking time for lunch, you will enable her to remain in control of her diabetes while helping you with your deadline.

Q. How can I tell if my work area is sensitive to the needs of those with diabetes?

A. To know if your work area is sensitive to the needs of employees, especially those with diabetes, you need to honestly assess your environment and organizational culture. To help you do this, complete the activity below, pretending to be a consultant hired to look at your work area from an outsider's perspective.

How can I help? Create a working environment that supports healthy lifestyle habits where people eat healthy, are physically active, and are able to manage their stress level. If you press employees to get more work done faster, setting unrealistic deadlines can affect their health.

Self-Assessment: Is My Work Environment Diabetes-Friendly?

Directions: Check the option that best describes your answer to the following questions about your work area. If a question doesn't pertain to your work environment, select "N/A" for "not applicable."

Part A: Work Environment

Within your work area, do people have

	Yes	No	Unsure	N/A
1. consistent work hours (nonrotating shifts)?	☐	☐	☐	☐
2. the ability to leave their work space whenever they need to?	☐	☐	☐	☐
3. the ability to set their own break and meal schedules?	☐	☐	☐	☐
4. sufficient time at breaks to attend to their diabetes needs?	☐	☐	☐	☐
5. the option of temporary work coverage by another coworker when recovering from a hypoglycemic episode?	☐	☐	☐	☐
6. access to meals/food at different times during the day?	☐	☐	☐	☐
7. the ability to select low-fat, low-calorie food from your company's cafeteria (if you have one)?	☐	☐	☐	☐
8. the ability to select low-fat, sugar-free food and beverages from vending machines?	☐	☐	☐	☐
9. access to a microwave and refrigerator at work?	☐	☐	☐	☐
10. adequate storage space to keep food refrigerated?	☐	☐	☐	☐

	Yes	No	Unsure	N/A
11. the ability to eat at their desk while working?	☐	☐	☐	☐
12. easy access to a bathroom or water fountain?	☐	☐	☐	☐
13. knowledge of who has diabetes in their work area and how to recognize hypoglycemia?	☐	☐	☐	☐
14. knowledge of what policy to follow if someone has hypoglycemia or a medical emergency?	☐	☐	☐	☐

Part B: Work Culture
Do people in your work area

	Yes	No	Unsure	N/A
15. keep candy dishes on their desk for people to snack on?	☐	☐	☐	☐
16. often bring in high-calorie treats to departmental functions, meetings, and break rooms?	☐	☐	☐	☐
17. often delay or skip lunch or breaks due to time conflicts and deadlines?	☐	☐	☐	☐
18. work much overtime in order to get their job done?	☐	☐	☐	☐

Part C: Corporate Environment
Does your company

	Yes	No	Unsure	N/A
19. offer health care benefits that include coverage for diabetes supplies and health education?	☐	☐	☐	☐
20. offer employee fitness or wellness programs?	☐	☐	☐	☐
21. offer diabetes-related support groups?	☐	☐	☐	☐
22. modify employee work areas so they are ergonomically safe?	☐	☐	☐	☐

	Yes	No	Unsure	N/A
23. follow one coordinated process for handling employee disabilities?	☐	☐	☐	☐
24. educate managers on how to report and handle disability issues?	☐	☐	☐	☐
25. offer short-term disability benefits to all employees?	☐	☐	☐	☐

> *Tallying your results:* The more "yes" responses you had for the work and corporate environment sections and "no" responses for the work culture section, the more friendly your work area is toward people with diabetes. If you checked "unsure" for some of the answers, you may wish to take a few minutes to investigate what the answers really are. If you discover your work area currently isn't diabetes-friendly, you may want to evaluate your answers to identify which areas you may want to make changes in to promote a more healthy, supportive environment for all your employees, not just the ones with diabetes.

Q. What type of diabetes benefits should I check to see if our employee medical insurance covers?

A. As a manager, you have the ability to ask your company's human resource department or benefits manager to review the different benefit options under your company's group insurance plan. If you do not have a group plan, you may want to ask your insurance agent about the insurance benefits for diabetes when your contract is renewed. Often, because no one asked if specific benefits were covered, they aren't always included—this is especially true in states where diabetes health benefits have not been mandated by law.

As a manager and diabetes advocate, you can help employees with diabetes request when contracts are renewed that diabetes health care benefits not be overlooked or lost. If you think the coverage is lacking, you can request that they discuss and clarify the coverage when negotiating contract renewals. Here are scenario examples of what to look for when reviewing health policies.

Scenario #1: Rick, your employee, was just diagnosed with type 2 diabetes and advised by his doctor to lose weight. He also needs to self-check his blood glucose level once a day. He has come to you with questions about his health care coverage. Do you know if your company's health plan includes:

- coverage for diabetes supplies?
- health education benefits so he can attend diabetes training programs or classes?
- health education benefits so he can work with a registered dietitian and learn how to modify his diet?
- benefits to help with weight loss?
- annual medical exams to have follow-up diabetes and eye care?

Scenario #2: Your employee Carol has had type 1 diabetes since she was a child and is under a lot of personal stress. Because her blood glucose control has been worsening, she would like to start intensive insulin therapy and learn how to cope with her stress. Do you know if her health plan includes:

- health education benefits to attend a class to learn how to manage her diabetes better?
- benefit coverage for an insulin pump and supplies?
- benefit coverage for blood glucose test strips, if she starts testing more than four times a day?
- easy access to doctors who specialize in diabetes?
- easy access to behavioral health specialists, psychologists, and social workers to help her learn to cope with stress?

Scenario #3: Your employee Lynn has had type 2 diabetes and high blood pressure for many years. Recently she's developed problems with her nerves, especially those in her feet. Her doctor has suggested she test her blood pressure at home and get a pair of orthopedic shoes that will provide more support to her feet than her current shoes do. Do you know if her health plan includes:

- benefit coverage for prescribed orthopedic shoes?
- benefit coverage for home blood pressure monitoring equipment?
- health education benefits so she can review her diet with a dietitian to help manage her blood pressure?

How can I help? Don't give out mixed signals. If you as a manager say you support people having healthy lifestyle habits, back up your words with the policies and resources they need to do it.

Q. I supervise Cathy, who has diabetes. How can I help her be the best worker she can be?

A. When trying to help an employee excel, it doesn't matter whether she has a medical condition (disability) or not. If you treat all people fairly and with respect, you can't go wrong.

When supervising or working with someone who has diabetes, share with her your honest interest and concern for their well-being. Because everyone's treatment plan for diabetes may be slightly different, ask her to explain how she cares for her diabetes (if she doesn't mind sharing this information with you). Find out if there are things or events in your work area that make it challenging for her to keep her blood glucose level controlled. The time and effort you invest in getting to know her will help make the worker feel appreciated and a valued part of your work family.

If you want to help your employee improve her work performance, you may decide to become a mentor or coach to her. Through coaching, you can help her gain the skills and knowledge to succeed at her job.

If you're thinking, "What? Me counsel or coach people? I don't know how to do that," don't worry. Learning how to motivate, counsel, or coach people is a skill you can learn with practice.

If you've avoided coaching people in the past because it felt awkward or scary, you're not alone. Common fears about being a coach or mentor are not knowing how to help or worrying about saying the wrong thing or giving bad advice. However, if you have a caring heart and want to see others succeed, as a manager you have a unique opportunity to help your employees.

Learning how to be a supportive manager and coach to your employees takes work and practice. To help you get started, here are five secrets to skillful coaching to remember when an employee seeks your help.

1. *Be a good listener.* Put your work aside and look directly at her when she talks. Don't try to write or work at your computer as you listen—it doesn't convey that you are really interested or sincere in your desire to listen or help. She will feel less important than your work. Practice patience and try not to interrupt as she talks. Refrain from offering advice or suggestions until she is done talking—often she will give you solutions to her problems if you give her time to talk aloud.

2. *Recognize what she's feeling (her emotions).* While she is talking, try to put yourself in her place. If she gets upset or angry or starts to cry, don't get scared—instead, acknowledge that you recognize what she is feeling. Doing this validates her emotions and offers you valuable insight into how strongly she feels about an issue or topic.

3. *Identify the problem by gathering all the facts.* Ask questions. Have her explain and clarify what the situation at hand is as she sees it. This will help you identify the problem more quickly and come up with options to resolve it. If you ask enough questions, you may even find that she is able to solve her own problems just by letting her talk out the situation in front of you! When she does that, you know you're being an effective coach.

4. *Define your role.* After identifying the situation or problem that the worker wants help with, take a few minutes to clarify with her the kind of help you can provide. Help her identify

other sources of help and support if she is unfamiliar with the available resources. If her problems are outside the scope of your job or ability, be honest and let her know she needs to look elsewhere. Be careful not to become a "fixer" who solves problems for her—she needs to learn to make her own decisions if she is going to gain the skills to problem-solve on her own.

5. *Help her make an action plan.* After identifying the problem, help her create an action plan to solve her problem. Help her list the steps she needs to take, goals to reach for, and resources she'll need. Let her implement her plan, and don't feel bad if she doesn't succeed at first. Learning from successes and failures is a process that's invaluable for revising goals and making future action plans.

To learn more about how to become a coach or counsel employees, you may want to explore some of the many books and audiotapes published on this topic, or you may want to attend classes and workshops taught through a local college or the company you work for to help polish your skills. Regardless of which method you choose, you'll soon learn that the counseling skills you gain are useful in all aspects of life—at home, work, and school.

How can I help? Become a good listener!

Q. How can I support Gerald, who works with me and takes insulin for his diabetes? As his manager, he's told me that he has diabetes. However, he hasn't told anyone else at work. I worry about him someday having an insulin reaction at work when I'm not around to help him. What should I do?

A. As it sounds as if you've already developed a good working relationship with your employee, ask him if he would meet with you to talk about your concerns. While you talk with him, practice your listening skills to identify his feelings about diabetes and why he hasn't told anyone else at work about it. Let him help you find a solution that is satisfactory to both of you.

To help you get a conversation going, here are some examples of questions you may want to ask him:

- Gerald, I really value the work you do for our company and enjoy working with you. However, I'm concerned about your diabetes. I worry that sometime you may have a low blood glucose level when you're at work and that I won't know how to help you. I'd feel more comfortable if I knew more about diabetes and how I can best support you. Can we talk about this for a few minutes?

- Gerald, you had mentioned to me that you take insulin to manage your diabetes. When do you take it? Is there a certain time that works best for you to take your lunch break so you can keep your diabetes under good control?

- Does anyone else here know that you have diabetes?

- If your blood glucose level ever got low, are you usually able to recognize it happening and treat yourself? Do you keep sugar in your desk or in a pocket for emergencies?

- When your blood glucose level is low, are there signs or symptoms that you'd have that I could recognize to know you may need help?

- When you have a low glucose level, do you feel okay to keep working, or would you like me to have someone cover your job for you until you're feeling better?

- In case you ever pass out from having a low blood glucose level, I'd feel more comfortable if we had an emergency plan set up so I'd know how to help you in the best way possible. Can we work on creating one together?

- I would hate for something bad to happen to you because nobody knew how to help you. I would feel more comfortable if at least two other people who work with you (besides me) know you have diabetes and could help you in an emergency. While I hope we would never need to use it, would it be all right if we created an emergency plan together so we know how to best help you?

Q. If I create an emergency plan for hypoglycemia with an employee, what should it include?

A. When creating emergency plans, check to see if there are existing plans already established where you work. While not all companies have them, it's nice when they are available through a human resources department so you don't have to create one by yourself. If no policy exists for handling medical emergencies at your company, here are things that you may wish to discuss with your diabetic employee and include in your plan.

> *How can I help?* As you create emergency plans, remember that the purpose is not to punish someone for having a low; rather, it's to ensure that the employee stays healthy and feels safe at work.

Emergency Hypoglycemia Plans

- Find out if he can tell when his blood glucose is getting low and whether he can treat himself or may need occasional help.

- If he takes insulin or diabetes pills, encourage him to always carry glucose tablets or a form of sugar in case he has an unexpected low and needs to self-treat.

- Decide if you should keep an emergency kit with glucose tablets somewhere in your work area that he can use to treat hypoglycemia for emergencies. Inform other managers in your area or at least one employee who works close by of where the kit is located and how to use it.

- Encourage him to routinely follow up with his health care provider for optimal care.

- Discuss if he is allowed to take bathroom or water fountain breaks, when needed.

- Encourage him to eat meals and breaks at scheduled times or allow him to be flexible scheduling his breaks.

- Give him advanced permission to quietly excuse himself during meetings at any time should he feel hypoglycemic.

(Some may feel embarrassed to do so and try to wait a low out, which could become dangerous.)

- Discuss if he can ask for temporary help covering his work if his blood glucose level drops and he doesn't feel well enough to do his job.

- Discuss whether he can monitor his blood glucose level where he works or needs to go to a restroom to do so.

- Discuss the health services and benefits he has to make sure he knows how to utilize available resources.

How can I help? Encourage employees to be physically active. If their job entails sitting for long periods of time, encourage them to take mini-walk or stretch breaks. Besides helping people with diabetes, it'll help all employees reduce stress, feel more alert and positive, and maintain high productivity levels.

Q. What should I do if a coworker or employee has an insulin reaction at work?

A. If you know that someone at work has diabetes and suspect that his blood glucose level is getting low, always start by asking if he feels all right. Remember, sometimes the symptoms may be due to reasons other than diabetes. If he confirms your suspicion that his blood glucose level is getting low, ask him if he has something to use as treatment, or would he like you to get him something. If he is conscious and able to treat himself, your role is to simply remain supportive and offer help if he asks for it. In most cases, he'll be able to treat himself quickly and effectively.

If the person you know with diabetes is conscious but unable to help himself due to low blood glucose, it's best to seek emergency professional help unless you've agreed ahead of time how to help him.

If you come across someone who has passed out, it's best to follow the emergency protocols established for your company. Unless you have a company nurse or emergency medical technician, this means that you'll probably need to call for outside emergency assistance (911). It's important to seek quick emergency help for him because you will probably be unsure what caused him to pass out. While it could be due to his diabetes, it may be a heart attack or something else.

Until emergency help arrives, if you or someone else on your staff is trained in emergency or basic life support skills, establish that he's breathing and help remove him from any immediate danger. You can gather the facts from bystanders to learn if anyone saw what happened and be ready to pass on the information to the emergency personnel when they arrive. If you suspect he could have passed out due to diabetes, you'll want to relay this information as quickly as possible.

How can I help? The best way to treat workplace hypoglycemia is to prevent it from happening. Encourage employees at risk of low blood glucose levels to always carry a form of sugar with them and to treat promptly. Remind them that taking care of their health is always a higher priority than finishing up on business.

Too many times when people have a hypoglycemic episode at work they'll share afterwards that they had felt the signs of a low blood glucose level. However, they either didn't have anything with them to treat the low, or what they had with them they didn't feel like eating, so in the process of going to get something to eat from a vending machine or from their desk, their blood glucose level dropped to the point where they ended up passing out.

Q. I work with Tim, who's had type 2 diabetes for ages. Over the past couple of months, though, he's been having problems keeping his blood glucose levels steady. It's starting to affect his work now. How can I, as a manager, help him?

A. Don't be afraid to share your observations and concerns with Tim. Explain to him how he's a good worker when his diabetes is in good control. However, when his blood glucose control is poor, you've noticed that it's affecting his work performance (for example, he's making mistakes, working more slowly, and having problems focusing on his work). Explain that you are concerned about him and his health and would like to offer your help to keep his diabetes under good control so he can keep feeling and working well.

Find out if he agrees with your observations and if he has any idea why his control has worsened over the past year. After you hear his thoughts, help him set up an action plan listing the steps he can take to improve his work performance by getting his diabetes back under control. Here are some troubleshooting ideas you could discuss with him if he needs help identifying where to start.

ENCOURAGING GOOD DIABETES CONTROL	
Possible Reasons for Poor Control	Steps to Take to Improve Diabetes Control
Decreased or increased activity level	Explore if his activity level has changed and ways he could get back on track if it's dropped
	Explore ways he could be more active at work if his job entails a lot of sitting
	If he's skipping his work breaks due to a high workload, remind him of the importance of taking his breaks and suggest ways he could use his breaks to be more active
Depression	Encourage him to talk with his doctor about how his mood affects his life and care for his diabetes
	Suggest that he talk with a counselor or therapist for help
Family problems	Suggest that he talk with a behavioral health counselor, social worker, or therapist for help
Illness other than diabetes	Encourage him to talk with his doctor to review his health status
	Encourage him to attend a health education class to learn more about his illness, if he's not sure how to care for his condition
Poor eating habits	Encourage him to talk with a registered dietitian to help him with his eating habits
Stress	Explore what could be causing the stress and ways to learn to cope with it
	Encourage him to enroll in a class to learn stress and/or time management skills
	If stress is due to personal problems, suggest he talk with a therapist or counselor through his health care provider or local church
Unknown causes	Encourage him to talk with his doctor or a diabetes specialist to review his diabetes treatment plan

Q. Does promoting good health care really have any effect on the work setting?

A. Yes. When employees feel good, they work their best. If someone's diabetes is poorly controlled, their productivity can be affected, as having either too high or low blood glucose levels can make people feel sluggish, affect their ability to think clearly, and cause mistakes. As one person with diabetes described it, "When my glucose level is out of control I feel like a space cadet and have trouble focusing on my work . . . when my diabetes is under good control, though, I give 110 percent to my job and am the best worker in my office."

The facts back this up. An exciting study published in 1998 by Harvard University researchers reported that people with type 2 diabetes who achieved good blood glucose control had less workplace absenteeism than those who had poor control. They also felt that their quality of life had improved, as did their level of productivity. So the answer as to how to reduce health care costs and improve work productivity is simply to encourage and support people with diabetes to have good diabetes control. It's a win-win situation for everyone!

How can I help?
Learn how employees around you care for their diabetes and encourage them to take care of their diabetes. Remind them that if their diabetes suffers, so will their work.

Q. A worker just reported to me that he thinks Dave is taking drugs, as he saw him using a syringe in the bathroom. Without violating Dave's confidence in me about his diabetes, how can I tell the rest of the staff that Dave has diabetes and isn't a drug user?

A. When someone spots another person using illegal drugs at work or anywhere, it's good to report it to someone in authority. Because Dave isn't using an illegal substance, there is no violation happening. However, people who don't know he has diabetes may start to wonder, and false rumors could start that could hurt his reputation.

In this situation, it's best to let Dave know what's going on. Explain to him that you know he's a great worker, but someone has expressed concern to you about seeing him inject himself in the bathroom. Because you want to protect his reputation and set minds at ease, ask him if others on staff know he has diabetes or if he's kept it a secret. If he's kept it a secret, reassure him that his diabetes won't change how you and others in your work family view him. To you, he's a great worker who just happens to have diabetes. However, because someone raised a concern that he may be doing something illegal, you'd like to set the record straight and stop any false rumors from getting started. Ask Dave if he would feel comfortable sharing with his work family that he has diabetes and takes insulin, or if it would be okay for you to share that information for him to the staff and the worker who reported him.

Chances are, if Dave has good diabetes control and has come to accept his condition, he'll have no problem telling others about his disease. He can be proud of how he cares for his health. If, however, he doesn't want people to know yet that he has diabetes, he may want to find a more private location when he takes his insulin.

Q. Our office always orders a cake to celebrate birthdays. Tomorrow is Marian's birthday, but I'm not sure if I should get a cake for her, since she has diabetes and can't eat sweets. What should I do?

A. If your office traditionally celebrates birthdays and special events, you may hurt Marian's feelings if you don't observe her birthday, even if your intentions are good. This would be another form of discrimination, if you treat her differently than everyone else is. Everyone likes to feel special on their birthday—Marian is no exception.

To help her feel like she's one of the office gang, it's important that her birthday is celebrated and recognized. Remember that it's the recognition that counts most—the cake is just how you decide to celebrate the recognition. So before you give up the thought of recognizing her birthday, ask her instead how she'd like the office to celebrate her special day. She's bound to feel honored that you care enough to ask her opinion and want only what's best for her health.

Given a choice, she may decide upon one of a couple options. First, she may decide that since her birthday happens only once a year, she'll eat a piece of cake. By planning ahead, she may want to incorporate a small piece of cake (a middle piece, not a corner piece with oodles of frosting) into her lunch meal and still keep her blood glucose level steady. On the other hand, she may suggest other things that could be used instead of cake to celebrate her birthday. Some simple ways to celebrate her birthday are listed below.

- special flavored coffee in the office coffeemaker (instead of regular coffee)
- biscotti or mini-muffins
- raw vegetables with a light dip to dunk them in
- assorted fresh fruit platters
- freshly popped popcorn
- root beer floats (use diet root beer and light or fat-free vanilla ice cream)
- cheerful balloons for her desk

Q. My boss has diabetes, and he often asks me to order lunch for him if he is going to be tied up in noon meetings. How do I know if I'm getting him the right things to eat to help him stay healthy?

A. The first thing you need to do is discuss with your boss what your responsibility is with his meals. Because he has a disease that is treated by diet, it's his responsibility to let you know what food to order and when he wants to eat it. It's also his responsibility to take time to eat on a regular basis. If he's asked you to order meals for him without giving you clear directions on what to order, that puts a lot of responsibility on your shoulders.

If he's asked you to obtain food for him, your responsibility is simply that of ordering the food and having it delivered by a specified time. If you order him food, it's up to him to eat it. But remember, you can't change his eating habits. Only he can. He is responsible for his health and his eating.

Next time you need to order his lunch, share your concern and interest in helping him eat and stay healthy. Explain how you'd like to be able to order the food he needs so he can focus on his work at the meetings and keep his diabetes under good control. If he hasn't shared what his meal plan is with you, ask him what he usually eats. Ask him what types of food and beverages he can and can't eat from the different restaurants you order food from. You can keep notes of the types of food he likes from different restaurants on file for reference when you order his meals. This way you will know what to order, and he will know he'll get the food he needs and wants to eat. He will also appreciate the attention and support you're giving him to cope with his disease. He may even ask you to keep notes on file about what important clients he works with like to eat. They'll be impressed with the attention they get, as it promotes high customer service when you go the extra mile to make sure they stay healthy, too.

Q. At work we sometimes have lunch meetings where food is catered in. Is there anything I should keep in mind when planning the meetings so that the environment is sensitive to the health needs of the attendees?

A. In the past, it was common for work meetings to include sweets or beverages. Now, in the age of fiscal responsibility, managers are evaluating more and more if treats are really needed for between-meal meetings. Many meetings are BYOB meetings (bring your own beverage or bring your own bag lunch), if attendees wish to sip on a cup of coffee or eat while discussing business.

When planning meetings, there are three simple rules to remember about menu planning. First, offer a variety of foods.

When planning the menu, use the food guide pyramid to offer attendees choices from all six food groups. This will ensure that everyone finds something they can eat and will be more satisfied with the food. Second, go easy on ordering high-fat items. Fried foods, meats with heavy sauces or gravies, and rich desserts that are high in fat can promote a feeling of satiety similar to eating a traditional Thanksgiving dinner. This can make people feel sluggish and crave a nap during afternoon meetings. By serving lower-fat foods, you may be pleasantly surprised at how ener- getic and productive your employees feel after lunch. Third, stick to your meeting agenda and serve meals promptly. If food is delayed because a meeting is running late, the person with diabetes may be at risk for a low blood glucose level. Appoint a meeting facilitator to keep the meeting on schedule, and if the meeting runs late excuse all who need to leave. This will allow the person with diabetes the opportunity to make a graceful exit out of the room to check the blood glucose level if they need to.

Q. Are there any tips or common courtesies I should remember so that I don't unintentionally offend someone who has diabetes?

A. When working with other people, having good manners is always important. Using good old-fashioned courtesy with col- leagues, employees, and customers helps create comfortable working relationships. Besides the general business etiquette rules of not shouting at people in meetings, returning phone calls promptly, being prompt, and showing up prepared for meetings, here are a few other tips to remember.

Diabetiquette

- Use the word *diabetic* as an adjective instead of a noun (e.g., *diabetic candy*). Don't call someone a diabetic. To be courteous (and more politically correct), refer to her as *someone who has diabetes.*

- Don't introduce a person with diabetes to others by blurting out, "This is Joe who has diabetes." Instead, introduce him in a way that makes him feel good about himself and lets others know what he does and how they may be working together in the future. For example, say, "This is Joe who works in marketing, and he does an awesome job handling the Acme account for us."

■ Don't break someone's confidence in you by talking about her medical status behind her back to others who don't need to know. Facts about her personal life should be considered private and confidential.

■ When planning meetings that include food, don't forget the dietary needs of the people attending and eating the food (e.g., low-fat, low-sugar, kosher, vegetarian).

■ Don't give employees candy and sweets on holidays or special occasions. They may not be able to eat it if they are trying to watch their diet to control their weight or take care of their health. Instead, offer healthy food like fruit baskets, flowers, or gift certificates to bookstores or restaurants, or consider hiring a masseuse for an afternoon to give everyone neck and shoulder massages. Now, those are treats everyone can enjoy!

Q. I'm an elementary school teacher and have a student, Diane, who has diabetes. What can I do to create a supportive school environment for my student to work in?

A. As a teacher, it's important for you to know that children with diabetes are protected under two federal laws to ensure that they receive education without discrimination. The Rehabilitation Act of 1973 (section 504) provides children with disabilities (e.g., diabetes) basic civil rights protection when enrolled in any program or activity that receives federal funding. The Individuals with Disabilities Education Act guarantees the right of disabled children to receive a free public education that includes special education and programming as needed. If you are unfamiliar with these two laws, you may wish to talk with your school's superintendent to learn more about the discrimination that has occurred against children with diabetes and other physical disabilities. Check to see what written policies exist in your school about diabetes.

As a teacher, work with the student's parents and your school's staff to agree upon an individualized education plan for how you can help the child manage his diabetes. The plan that you come up with may include guidelines for :

- treating hypoglycemia and how the guidelines will be shared with his other teachers (regular or substitute ones who cover for you on your days off)

- eating or not eating snacks in class, depending upon his needs

- going to the bathroom or water fountain when he needs to

- testing his blood glucose level when needed (agree if he can do this in the classroom or if he needs to go to the principal or nurse's office to do it)

- participating in school activities, including recess, physical education class, and afterschool sports

- being out sick more often than other children

- scheduling more frequent parent/teacher conferences for the parents to stay updated on their child's progress

CHAPTER 7

Understanding My
Emotions . . . to Better
Cope with Their Diabetes

I WAS STUNNED WHEN I HEARD THE NEWS MY WIFE HAD DIABETES. WE HAD
GONE TO SEE HER DOCTOR BECAUSE SHE FELT TIRED ALL THE TIME AND HAD A
SORE ON HER FOOT THAT WASN'T HEALING. WE NEVER EXPECTED TO BE TOLD SHE
HAD DIABETES. I NEVER IMAGINED ALL THE LIFESTYLE CHANGES WE'D NEED TO
MAKE. I STILL FEEL LIKE I'M ADJUSTING TO IT, AND IT'S BEEN ALMOST A YEAR!

Shock. Disbelief. Fear. Do you remember how you first felt
when you learned that a friend or loved one had diabetes? You
may have found yourself asking, "You've got what?" or "How do
they know? They must have gotten the tests wrong!" You probably felt a range of emotions, from denial to fear. If you weren't
familiar with what diabetes is, you may have even wondered if
you'd get it, too, or if you did something that may have caused
it. Or you may know someone who has developed complications
from diabetes—lost a limb, lost their sight, or developed heart
problems—and fear what could happen to him. Diabetes can
feel scary.

When someone gets diabetes or any serious medical condition, it's common to feel uncertain at first and wonder what it all
means. Even though it happened to someone else, the effect of
his diabetes has the potential to reach everyone close to him—
including you! At first the diagnosis may seem overwhelming
and even complex as you try to grasp an understanding of what
diabetes is and how it's treated. The more you learn, you may
feel powerless at first as you realize that while you'd love to fix
things and make him feel better, you can't. As he starts to adopt

190

new lifestyle habits, you may feel compelled to change some of your habits too, even though you hadn't planned on it or wanted to. You may have a sense that you've lost something and things will never be the same again. If it's a family member or spouse with diabetes, you may even feel that you've lost your dream of having a "normal" family as the reality of coping with a chronic illness hits your home. However, that can also lead you to ponder what "normal" families are in the first place.

Serious health conditions like diabetes or heart disease have the ability to act as a catalyst to either bring people closer together or promote tension that drives them apart. The direction it takes depends a lot on whether the people involved have the coping skills needed to handle the emotions they feel and adjust to the changes diabetes can bring to someone's lifestyle.

How has diabetes affected your life? While people with diabetes are often asked this question, it's not always asked of the family and friends around them. This chapter will help you assess the impact diabetes has had on your life and identify your emotions. You'll learn about positive coping skills and ideas on how to build a supportive environment for both you and the person with diabetes. Let's start by taking the quiz below.

Quiz: How Does Diabetes Affect Me?

Directions: For each question below, check the box that best describes your response. Be honest with your feelings. You can check more than one box for each question and write in additional emotions if the responses provided do not adequately describe what you feel. (*Note:* For consistency, the person with diabetes in the questions will be referred to as *he* or *him*.)

1. When you first learned that he had diabetes, how did the news make you feel?
   ☐ relieved   ☐ overwhelmed
   ☐ hopeful   ☐ shocked
   ☐ betrayed   ☐ angry
   ☐ concerned   ☐ other: _____

2. How do you feel about his diabetes today?

- [ ] grateful
- [ ] angry
- [ ] frustrated
- [ ] ashamed
- [ ] hopeful
- [ ] afraid
- [ ] confident
- [ ] other: _____

3. When you think about his future with diabetes, how do you feel?

- [ ] worried
- [ ] scared
- [ ] anxious
- [ ] accepting
- [ ] neutral
- [ ] helpless
- [ ] hopeful
- [ ] other: _____

4. When you think about your future with him, how do you feel?

- [ ] worried
- [ ] grateful
- [ ] afraid
- [ ] depressed
- [ ] optimistic
- [ ] anxious
- [ ] realistic
- [ ] other: _____

5. When he has a low blood glucose level (hypoglycemia), how do you feel?

- [ ] afraid
- [ ] calm
- [ ] helpless
- [ ] respectful
- [ ] annoyed
- [ ] confident
- [ ] embarrassed
- [ ] other: _____

6. When you see him eating foods that aren't good for him, how do you feel?

- [ ] angry
- [ ] worried
- [ ] ambivalent
- [ ] happy
- [ ] accepting
- [ ] guilty
- [ ] sad
- [ ] other: _____

7. When you try to help your friend control his diabetes, how do you feel?

☐ appreciated   ☐ ignored

☐ guilty   ☐ anxious

☐ confident   ☐ happy

☐ powerless   ☐ other: _____

Results: Because everyone has a right to have and feel emotions, there are no right or wrong answers to any of the questions. Your feelings are real and unique to you. However, take a moment to look back at the emotions you checked. Do you see any patterns or trends in them? Did you mark mostly positive or negative feelings? Or did you mark a mixture of positive and negative feelings?

If you feel that your answers were mostly positive, you have learned to successfully cope with a friend or loved one having diabetes. While this doesn't mean that you won't get angry or worried once in a while, it does show that you're not letting diabetes dominate your relationship. On the other hand, if your responses were mostly negative or you wished they more positive, it means that diabetes is having an effect on your life. It's up to you to decide now if you want that effect to continue, or if you want to change it.

Q. I'm not used to talking about my feelings. I was taught when growing up that emotions were a sign of weakness. Were other people taught this, too?

A. Yes. For years, many cultural groups have valued the ability to keep one's emotions to oneself. Emotions were viewed as disruptive and socially unacceptable. Have you ever heard someone say, "Keep a smile on your face and don't let anyone see you're crying on the inside"? Or how about, "If you're frustrated, angry, or feeling sad, just get over it," "Keep a stiff upper lip," "Try to think about their feelings instead of your own"? Or, "It is okay to know about your feelings, just not to show them. This can cause internal stress. Because of these beliefs and values, over time many people have learned to bottle up or stuff their feelings inside, keeping them private.

In our society, showing and expressing emotion has typically been more acceptable for women than men. Often, showing public displays of affection or emotions was viewed in the past as a moral weakness or as a troublesome behavior to be avoided. Children were taught by parents to remain calm and avoid emotional outbursts. This belief is even evident in games and sports, where often the best players are those who are able to hide their emotions, keeping a focused expression. This is shown in the advice to "keep a straight face" when playing poker or "stay calm, cool, and collected" when negotiating in the business world. However, this view has started to change.

> *Did you know . . . feelings don't make you weak, repressing them does.*

In recent years, researchers have been studying the purpose of emotions, and what they've found is enlightening. Emotions play an important role in how we communicate with others and make decisions. Our emotions or "gut instinct" helps us make intelligent decisions where logic alone can't. Business leaders value people who are aware of their emotions and can sense them in others. Employees who show strong emotions (are friendly, enthusiastic, proud of their work, caring, and trustworthy) and have developed strong people skills are highly prized in the workplace, as they relate well with customers. This makes them more effective at their job, as without emotions, employees wouldn't know if their decisions were morally right or wrong or how to please their customers.

Emotions help us experience life in all its richness and diversity. According to Daniel Goleman in his book *Emotional Intelligence*, emotions help prepare our bodies to respond to situations and changes that occur throughout each day. When we feel afraid, our bodies automatically prepare to take action, to run away or to fight. Emotions such as pain, anger, and intense sadness can signal to us that there is something wrong in our life. Research has show that many negative emotions—stress, anxiety, anger, and depression—can lead to physical symptoms, poor lifestyle behaviors, and negative health status. However, when we feel happy or loved, our bodies relax and feel good about life. Goleman suggests that the more we can become aware of our emotions, the more we can learn to harness their energy and manage them in positive ways. We could even use our emotions to motivate ourselves and those around us to lead healthy lifestyles.

Q. What emotions do people usually feel when someone they care about gets diabetes?

A. When someone close to you is first diagnosed with diabetes, it's common to feel shocked. It may feel as if you had the rug snatched out from under your feet, causing you to fall to the floor. In a flash, you realize that you're looking at the world in a totally different way than you were just moments ago, because you're sitting on the floor looking up at people and things. You search around for answers as to what may have caused you to fall. A mixture of emotions—pain, embarrassment, anger, or humor—may wash over you as you come to accept the fact that while you're still on the floor, you are unhurt. To get your life back in order, you organize your thoughts, polish off your self-image, and return to doing your usual activities. Life goes on.

Just as you'd respond and recover from slipping on a rug, you will feel a mixture of emotions after the shock of diagnosing diabetes wears off. The feelings you may experience can include grief, even though you yourself don't have diabetes. For instance, you can feel a sense of loss of all the expectations and dreams you used to have with the person who has diabetes. You may suddenly feel vulnerable as you realize your own mortality. You may grieve over the loss of lifestyle habits you used to share. These losses are real and need to be recognized. The grief needs to be coped with.

Elizabeth Kübler-Ross, in her work in the 1960s and 1970s with hundreds of terminally ill adults and children, identified that while people grieve in different ways, most go through five stages of grief as they learn to cope with their loss of physical health, life, and lifestyle behaviors: denial, anger, bargaining, depression, and acceptance. How fast people go through the stages varies from person to person. Some people can even get stalled in different stages for years. How fast you move through the stages may be faster or slower than for the person you know with diabetes. You each need to go through them at your own pace.

As people grieve, denial is the first stage people go through. It's recognized by reactions of "No, that can't be true!" "The doctor must be wrong, how could you have diabetes?" For most people, this stage is quickly followed by the second stage, anger and fear. During anger, the classic reaction is to wonder "Why?" "How did this happen?" "It's not fair!" During this stage, you may try to find something or someone to blame because you feel helpless. At some point, anger turns into bargaining, the third stage. Bargaining is when you initially start thinking about making lifestyle changes but aren't sure the benefit of changing is worth it. You may catch yourself saying, "If I just cook his food so it's low in fat and sugar, then I've done my part. The rest of the family and I don't need to eat his food because it's not our problem." But bargaining only works for a while, until you start to understand that this diabetes isn't going to go away. It's permanent. This leads to the fourth stage, depression, where you experience a feeling of sadness as you mourn the loss of some of your hopes, dreams, and old way of life. Once you go through this stage, you can reach the final stage, acceptance. You learn to accept the fact that your life has gone through change, but you also start to see the possibilities ahead. You may even feel excitement at new opportunities that may arise and feel stronger from the experience you just went through.

Did you know . . . just because you don't have diabetes doesn't mean that you can't feel its emotional effects.

Q. Is it possible to ever stop feeling overwhelmed by diabetes?

A. With time, yes. It's common when someone first learns about diabetes to feel overwhelmed by it and the lifestyle changes it may require. However, with time, most learn to adjust and adopt new habits that feel natural a couple of years later. Some even report feeling grateful for the role diabetes played in their lives to motivate them to lead healthier lifestyles than before. Diabetes caused them to reflect on what they wanted from life and even inspired them to pursue dreams and activities they otherwise may not have. Because the lifestyle for diabetes is healthy, entire families report they are eating healthier and are often surprised at how satisfied they feel eating more fresh fruits and vegetables and consuming less fat in their diets. They enjoy being more physically active because it energizes them, reduces stress, and allows them to enjoy the company of friends through walking and exercising together. For this reason, many people report appreciation for the good things that happened in their lives because of diabetes.

If you're feeling overwhelmed by diabetes, you need to continue learning more about it and give yourself time to adjust. If you feel that you have to give up all your favorite things because of someone else's diabetes, stop and think for a moment about what you are really giving up. Is it eating unlimited amounts of sweets or high-calorie foods? Is it watching unlimited amounts of television and using a remote control to change channels? Is it skipping meals instead of eating three meals a day? If this sounds familiar, ask yourself what shape you will be in ten or twenty years if you continue your habits—will you be healthy? What will you look like? Will you be able to do everything you want to do?

The lifestyle habits people with diabetes adopt are the very habits everyone should follow, young and old alike. We can all benefit from them and feel positive when we have them. The only difference is that people with diabetes need healthy habits to keep their diabetes under control. You, on the other hand, can choose if and when you want to do it. When you come to accept diabetes as neither a curse nor a shameful condition, you can start to find the positive aspects of living a healthy lifestyle.

Remember, it's not his fault he got diabetes. No one is to blame. However, he is responsible for dealing with his condition. You get to decide if you want to support him or not.

Q. How can I learn to cope with the negative emotions and feelings I have about diabetes?

A. While there are many emotions you may feel, you may find that only a few bother you to the point where you want to do something about them. Emotions are a way your body reacts to situations around you. So to cope with or change how you feel, you need to start by first identifying what emotion you're feeling and what could be triggering or causing it.

Because many of us have been taught to stuff our negative emotions deep down inside us or ignore them, at first it may be hard and feel a bit uncomfortable to recognize what you're feeling. Therefore, the first place to start is by acknowledging to yourself that it's okay to have feelings, it's normal and nothing to feel ashamed of. Emotions are a part of what makes you a unique person and help you value what is important in your life. Ignoring or wishing your feelings would just go away or bottling them up inside you creates internal stress and fails to resolve what is causing the emotion.

Once you put a name to how you're feeling (e.g., happy, sad, mad, or flustered), identify how you usually react to that emotion. For example, pretend someone smashed into your car, denting the passenger-side door. How would you feel and first react? Would you feel angry and react by saying something under your breath? Would you shout at the person who hit your car? Would you cry or laugh? Would you hold in your anger and politely (through gritted teeth) ask for the name of his insurance company? Or would you do something else? The reaction you identified is one method you currently use to cope with feelings of anger.

Is there a right or wrong reaction to have? Yes. Depending upon the culture you were brought up in and the societal values where you live, some reactions are socially unacceptable. For example, if you respond to anger by harming yourself or others around you, that is a form of abuse—verbal, physical, or emotional—and is not socially accepted as an appropriate reaction. While venting (talking or cussing without candor) was previously recommended by therapists as a way to cope with anger, recent studies are showing that venting may only increase feelings of aggression. To defuse anger, more effective reactions to use include relaxation techniques (deep breathing and counting to ten before responding to what is angering you), exercise, distraction (doing something else that is calming, enjoyable, and forces your mind to think of something else), and humor.

As children, we learn from our parents and friends how to cope with our emotions. We learn that it's okay to clap our hands, whistle, or hum when we feel happy. We learn that it's not correct to hit people when we get mad or whine when we feel life is unfair. When feelings make us feel uncomfortable, we learn ways to cope to make them go away. While some coping methods are effective, others are not. For example, some people cope with emotions and stress by overeating, drinking alcohol, or smoking cigarettes. While this allows the person to escape from the feeling for a few minutes, the emotion quickly returns, as the trigger causing it hasn't been dealt with.

What methods do you use to cope with emotions? Complete the quiz below to help you identify how you react to your feelings. Be honest and answer what first comes to your mind.

Quiz: How Am I Coping? A Self-Assessment

Directions: From the list of coping methods that follows, select the response(s) that best completes each question. Write your response in the blanks provided. You can use a response more than once.

1. When I feel angry, I _____.

2. When I feel afraid, I _____.

3. When I feel stressed, I _____.

4. When I feel bored, I _____.

5. When I feel happy, I _____.

6. When I feel sad, I _____.

7. When I'm not in control of a situation, I feel _____.

Coping Methods

- act outrageously
- bite my fingernails
- blame others
- call a friend to talk
- clean my room or house
- deny or ignore my feelings
- distract myself by doing something else
- drink alcohol or pop
- eat food or sweets
- exercise
- grit my teeth
- hit something
- laugh
- let other people take over
- practice deep breathing
- practice positive self-talk
- practice visualization techniques
- set priorities
- shop (spend money)
- shout or cuss
- smoke tobacco
- try to think logically
- use drugs
- wish the feelings away
- withdraw

Results: There are many ways to cope with feelings. Look back at your answers. Do you think the ways you currently use are effective or ineffective? Do the methods you use harm yourself or anyone else?

If you think you may be coping in a negative or ineffective way, it is possible to learn new skills, to change the reactions you use. While it takes hard work and time, learning to use positive coping skills will help you feel more in control, less trapped, and more self-confident. Remember, you have the ability and control to choose how to cope with your emotions.

1. *Recognize what you're feeling.* Be honest with yourself and put a name to the emotion you're feeling. Don't be ashamed of your feelings or try to minimize them; they are real and need to be felt and shared. But, don't confuse feelings with thoughts. While thoughts are what you think and contemplate, feelings consist of what you sense or perceive. For example, if you "thought" someone stole your car, you may "feel" angry or puzzled.

   While recognizing feelings may feel uncomfortable at first, remember that your emotions serve a purpose and help your body deal with what happens to you throughout your day. Being aware of emotions is the first step in learning how to manage them.

2. *Stop to think before you react.* After you recognize the emotion you're feeling, try to halt what you're doing. Try not to react to the emotion right away. Instead, take a step backwards (mentally) to evaluate what your first instinct was for handling the emotion. Decide whether the coping method you were about to use would have been effective. Would it have resolved the emotion and dealt with the trigger? Could it have hurt someone else? By catching yourself to stop and think about your response, you will help prevent yourself from saying or doing something you may regret later. Stopping before reacting allows you the chance to change your mind.

3. *Take control—choose how you want to express and cope with your feelings.* If you feel mad, it's okay to stamp your foot. If you feel like crying, go right ahead and cry. But if you're happy, go ahead and laugh, smile, or give someone a hug. Choose how you want to react. If you haven't shared your feelings and concerns about diabetes with the person who has it, schedule some time to sit down together and talk about it. Let her know how her diabetes is affecting you, and try to find solutions to resolve your feelings. Be careful not to blame the person with diabetes; she can't help having it. If you have trouble putting your feelings into words, consider writing them out in

a journal or talking to a friend. For additional guidance, you may want to talk with a professional counselor for individualized assistance learning new coping skills or join a support group. Effective Coping Strategies (below) lists ways to cope with negative feelings in a productive way.

4. *Check your attitude—think positively.* When you're in the midst of a difficult situation, remember that how you respond is what matters the most. Check your attitude toward what's going on. You have the ability to decide how you want to react. If you think good thoughts about yourself (and others) and what you can do, you'll start to believe that there are wonderful things ahead of you in life to explore. If you don't, life can look overwhelming, bleak, and lonely.

Effective Coping Strategies

- Exercise—be physically active to channel your energy.
- Check the facts before reacting (think logically and see if there are reasons for why something happened that you're not aware of yet).
- Distract yourself—do something fun and relaxing.
- Call up a friend to talk and get a second opinion.
- Laugh or cry.
- Listen to your favorite music.
- Meditate.
- Practice deep-breathing exercises.
- Practice positive self-talk.
- Relax with a favorite hobby.
- Read an inspirational or self-help book.
- Smile.
- Spend time with a pet.
- Take a walk outdoors.
- Volunteer to help someone.
- Watch your favorite comedy show or movie.
- Write down your thoughts in a journal.

Q. Some days I feel so helpless. I wish I could better help my husband, who has diabetes, and fix things so that he didn't have to take insulin anymore. Sometimes I'm afraid to leave him alone in case he needs something to eat or has a low. How can I get rid of this feeling?

A. When you care about someone who is trying to cope with an illness or medical condition, it's normal to want to make him feel better. However, diabetes isn't like a scraped knee that you can bandage up and fix. Diabetes has no cure and requires constant attention to control.

When caring for someone starts to feel as though your life is wrapped up solely around him and his needs, you have crossed the line from caring to overcaring. Caring for someone doesn't mean taking over his life and making all his decisions for him—that's called overcaring. When you do this, you've tried to take control of the situation. You've become a caretaker. Being a caretaker to someone who doesn't want one can have a negative effect on your relationship. In addition, allowing someone to not take full responsibility for his disease and letting you be their caretaker doesn't promote a healthy relationship either. Instead, it can result in a type of dysfunctional codependency. When overcaring for someone results in you not having the time or energy to care for your own health, you need to reassess your role and responsibility in the relationship.

While it's natural to want to care for someone you love, you need to recognize where your responsibility starts and ends. In Rhoda Levin's book *Heartmates: A Guide for the Spouse and Family of the Heart Patient,* she explains how women in our culture learn at early ages to be caretakers or nurturers. We play "house" and model roles

> *Did you know . . . you have the ability to choose how you want to cope with your emotions. To do so, you need to: 1) identify how you feel; 2) stop to think before you react; 3) choose how you want to express your feelings; and 4) check your attitude—think positively.*

after our parents. To feel successful as a caretaker, we learn we need to protect our spouse and children from harm. However, that isn't always possible, especially when trying to deal with a chronic disease that has no cure. Consequently, as a caregiver you may occasionally feel helpless, which can prompt you to cross the line from caring to overcaring in an effort to take control of the situation. If you take on the responsibility for your spouse's feelings and actions, he can become dependent on you. He may feel he's even lost his independence. At the same time, you run the risk of feeling resentful of the care you feel you need to give him.

If you feel helpless about your husband's diabetes, you need to look at how you and your husband are sharing the responsibility of his disease. To do this, first acknowledge the fact that you cannot fix his diabetes or make it go away; that's out of your control. Second, acknowledge that your husband is ultimately responsible for making decisions about what he wants to do or not do with his life. When he chooses to do something you disagree with, you can't take responsibility for his actions or nag him to change. Only he can change. Third, assess with your husband what help he wants and needs from you versus what he is able to do on his own. Be realistic. If he's physically able to care for himself, don't treat him like an invalid or like he's made out of glass and will break. Don't pamper him. Instead, help your spouse learn to care for himself so that you will feel more confident taking time for yourself and your needs. This will help ease your worry that you need to always be there for him.

If, however, he is physically unable to care for himself, know when to ask for help caring for him. Discuss between the two of you and with your family and a health care provider or counselor what your responsibility is and when it's okay to ask for outside help.

> *Did you know . . .*
> caring for someone
> doesn't mean taking
> over his life and
> making all his
> decisions for him.

Quiz: Am I an Overcaring Person?

Directions: Place a checkmark next to the response that best answers each question. (*Note:* For consistency, the person with diabetes in each question is referred to as *she* or *her*.)

	Yes	No	Unsure
1. Do you listen at night when she gets up to go to the bathroom?	☐	☐	☐
2. Do you sometimes stay awake at night listening to her breathe to make sure she's okay?	☐	☐	☐
3. Do you feel tired after a night's sleep?	☐	☐	☐
4. Do you avoid foods you like to eat because of her diet?	☐	☐	☐
5. Do you help her test her blood glucose level and record her results in her logbook?	☐	☐	☐
6. Do you feel personally responsible when she doesn't follow her diet?	☐	☐	☐
7. When you are at a doctor's appointment with her, do you feel responsible for how well her diabetes is under control?	☐	☐	☐
8. Have you stopped doing things you used to enjoy before she got diabetes?	☐	☐	☐

Results: If you answered "yes" or "unsure" to most of the questions above, you may have crossed the line from caring to overcaring. To know for sure, review the role each of you are playing in caring for her diabetes and how her diabetes is affecting your life.

Q. I can't get over this guilty feeling that I may have caused my daughter's diabetes. Do you think she could have gotten it from the food I cooked?

A. While it's common for parents to want to blame themselves for their child's diabetes, people do not get diabetes from the food or candy they eat. Neither worrying nor thinking bad thoughts causes it. Even though you may have a family history of diabetes, you personally didn't cause her diabetes—genetic and family traits are out of your control. The guilty feelings you are having are more likely due to a desire to find a reason—something concrete—to explain why it happened. In your mind, you may be trying to find something to blame to help you cope with the situation. As you search for a reason, you may imagine different "what-if" scenarios, wondering what would have happened if you had noticed her illness sooner, cooked different foods, stopped her from eating so many cookies, or done something else. You may even wonder if her diabetes was due to your family's genetics or your spouse's. But because you can't find a perfect answer, questions and scenarios keep replaying in your mind, giving you this uneasy feeling.

When a family member is afflicted with diabetes, it's common for parents and family members to experience feelings of guilt or shame. While these feelings are uncomfortable, they can also be helpful if you use them as a catalyst to reflect back on what happened and honestly question yourself as to whether you really could be responsible for her diabetes. When you consider all the facts, you'll soon realize that the end result (her getting diabetes) would have happened regardless of whether you cooked spaghetti instead of meat loaf for supper or baked fewer cookies. This is true because research tells us that diabetes doesn't happen overnight, it develops over time—years—for reasons we still don't understand.

For your own health and well-being, it's not good to focus on the past, feeling guilty and spending countless hours pondering "what-ifs" and "should-have" thoughts about something that was out of your control. It's not productive. Instead, learn to accept the fact that your daughter has diabetes and no one was to blame, neither you nor her. While you can't turn back the clock, you can look forward and help your daughter cope with her disease. You can support her and the rest of your family's efforts to live a healthy lifestyle by living for the future. Have confidence in all the wonderful things you have done and still do as a parent. Be there for her, taking the time to listen to her feelings. This will help you regain a positive focus on your life and hers.

Did you know . . . when you live with guilt, you live in the past, reflecting on all the "what-ifs" and " should-haves" you could have done. However, when you accept that diabetes can happen to good people, you live in the present and think about what you can do.

Q. I get so frustrated with my wife. She has type 1 diabetes and never seems to be able to keep her blood glucose levels in her target range. I hear other people with diabetes say they always have readings in their target range. Is it harder for some people to keep their diabetes under control? What can I do?

A. Yes. Depending upon the type of diabetes people have and how it's treated, some people have an easier time than others keeping their blood glucose readings in their target goal range. This is most commonly true of people with type 2 diabetes who are able to manage their disease without taking insulin because their pancreas is still able to produce it. However, even these people will notice that their glucose readings fluctuate. This is because there are many factors that affect glucose levels (such as medication, food, exercise level, and illness) and cause the level to naturally waver within a certain range. It's uncommon for a person to have the same glucose level every single time it is checked.

As you help your wife interpret her glucose levels, think about her target blood glucose range as a bull's-eye that she's aiming for to achieve good diabetes control. With practice tracking her glucose readings, she will be able to anticipate whether her blood glucose levels will be high, low, or near her target range, depending upon how consistent she is with her diet, activity level, and general state of health. When she has a blood glucose reading within target range, she scores a bull's-eye. When she's a little above or below her target, she's close, which isn't bad. Depending on her insulin regimen, she can learn to possibly adjust her insulin dose to bring her blood glucose level back in range before the next time she tests. If occasionally she has a glucose reading that is way out of target range that she can't account for, she'll need to watch carefully over the next couple of days to see if the reading repeats itself. If a pattern emerges, she should talk with her health care provider to discuss if her treatment program needs adjustment. If no pattern emerges, then she can chalk up the reading as a fluke.

Remember, keeping diabetes under good control takes a lot of work and effort. People who use insulin as a treatment method will experience more variation in their numbers, so expecting blood glucose readings to always be within a target range is unrealistic.

A recent study at the Barbara Davis Center for Childhood Diabetes at the University of Colorado revealed that adults with type 1 diabetes who had excellent glucose control (HbA1c levels below 7%) had blood glucose readings within their target only half of the time. This was with a target range of 70–150 mg/dl. What this tells us is that target ranges are just what they sound like, a target to aim for. While sometimes the readings may be higher or lower, the goal is to keep the blood glucose level as near or within the target range as much as possible while avoiding overly high or low readings.

Did you know . . . people with type 1 diabetes who have excellent blood glucose control have glucose readings within their target range only roughly half the time.

Q. I wish we could go out and visit friends like we used to. Ever since my wife got diabetes, we've had to stay home instead of dining out because she's afraid she won't find the right food to eat. Is this how it's going to be for the rest of our married life?

A. When someone is first diagnosed with diabetes, it's normal for her to feel nervous about eating away from home, as she's leaving a safe environment where she has control over when and what she eats and enters one full of uncertainties. However, with practice most people find that they can enjoy dining out with friends and family as they become familiar with their diet for diabetes. If your wife is unsure of what to eat or select when dining out, encourage her to talk with a registered dietitian who specializes in diabetes or a certified diabetes educator. They can teach both of you how to adjust for different situations that may occur when dining out, traveling, and visiting friends. By learning how to plan ahead for challenging situations, she will gain confidence in her ability to adjust her food choices or schedule appropriately.

For support, consider joining a local diabetes support group. Through meeting other people with diabetes, you and your wife can meet other people going through the same experience— learning how to cope with diabetes. From them, you can learn many valuable tips on how to successfully manage diabetes on a day-to-day basis.

In the meantime, you can help her adjust and start enjoying socializing with friends again by inviting some of your closest friends to visit you at your home, where your wife feels most comfortable. Enlist the aid of your friends to invite you, in return, to their house, explaining your wife's concerns and diet needs. If they're good friends, they'll be glad to help create a safe environment in their home for your wife to visit and enjoy a pleasant meal. As she gains confidence that she can socialize outside your home, soon you'll become social butterflies again.

Q. I am so frustrated with my husband. He uses his diabetes as an excuse when he wants to get out of doing something he doesn't want to do. How can I get him to do the things that I want to do sometimes?

A. When one person wants something different than someone else, the situation can result in tension. This tension is caused by differences in each other's personal values and goals. To resolve the tension, start by clariying what the troublesome behavior is that is causing the tension and identify possible solutions to resolve the tension. Then, schedule a quiet time with your husband to calmly discuss (not argue or overreact) the concern you have and what you see is the problem causing it.

As you talk, try to understand his point of view. Confront him politely and ask him to clarify why he can't do something because of his diabetes. You may find out that he could be feeling anxious about having hypoglycemia or eating out in public. He may not be sure how to manage his diabetes in new situations. By understanding his reasons, you'll be able to work together to create solutions you both feel comfortable with. You may even be surprised at what you learn through the process and find that your relationship is strengthened because you'll understand each other better.

However, if he doesn't have a good reason for why he can't do something because of his diabetes, you've called his bluff. You've confirmed that diabetes isn't the real reason why he doesn't want to do something— it's just an excuse he uses because it's worked in the past to get his way. It's up to you to decide if you want him to continue using his condition as an excuse. If you don't, you'll need to sit down and discuss what he and you would like to do and compromise to find a solution that's agreeable to both of you. This may include doing things sometimes without him.

> *Did you know . . . those who seek to understand why people have different opinions and beliefs find new ways to build supportive relationships.*

Q. I worry that my spouse will get complications from diabetes someday. Is it normal to feel this way?

A. Yes. Worrying about a loved one who has diabetes is a common feeling spouses have. A survey by the American Diabetes Association of nearly 2,000 spouses of people with diabetes revealed that 58 percent worry about their spouse developing diabetic complications later in life. Of these people, over half (56%) worried about their spouse dying, 27 percent felt guilty that they should be doing more to help them manage their diabetes, and 22 percent were angry and felt that their spouse should be doing more to care for their diabetes.

While it's normal to wonder about the future, another finding from the survey was that almost half of the people surveyed didn't worry about their spouse developing complications. Worry is really a form of fear and anxiety that happens when our imagination and emotions take control of our thoughts. However, worry can be calmed through faith, hope, and trust in yourself and others. When your "worry" voice starts speaking to you, learn to confront your negative thoughts with the facts about diabetes. Distract yourself by doing something else— think about what's positive in your life, whistle a song, pray, take a walk—so that your thoughts stay positive. Worry over loved ones can be lessened when you channel your thoughts away from the many things that could happen and take action to make sure they are receiving the treatment that they need to care for their disease. Because worry doesn't solve anything, focus your energy on what you can do today. Enjoy each day for what you have instead of worrying about what may never happen.

Q. Ever since my father was diagnosed with diabetes, he's been really moody. I think maybe he's depressed because he's had to give up everything he likes to eat and do. How can I help him?

A. When people are adjusting to changes in lifestyle, whether it's with their family, at work, or with their health, it's common for them to feel a variety of emotions. These feelings can range from happiness to sadness. However, when the sad feelings start to last longer than two weeks and combine with feelings of help-lessness, hopelessness, anxiety, apathy, or irritability, more may be happening than just common grief. These symptoms can be a signal of depression.

Depression is an illness that is more than feeling sad. It's a serious condition that can affect a person's feelings, thoughts, and behaviors, causing mood swings. When it occurs in some-one with diabetes, it can cause him to stop taking his medication, following his diet (e.g., over- or undereating), and exercising. Consequently, his blood glucose control worsens, which can result in either hypoglycemia or hyperglycemia.

While researchers are still trying to find out what triggers depression, people with diabetes or who have a family history of depression are at risk for developing it. When depression devel-ops, a chemical imbalance occurs in a person's body that results in the variety of symptoms that a person may have. What distin-guishes depression from simple sadness is that the feelings per-sist over weeks and combine with four or more other symptoms (see Symptoms of Depression on page 213). Because many of the symptoms of depression are similar to that of poor diabetes control, depression is unfortunately often overlooked and undertreated in people with diabetes. It's estimated that only one out of three people with depression receives treatment that can improve their quality of life. This is unfortunate as there are a number of treatment options available, ranging from med-ications to psychotherapy, that could be used to help them feel better.

If you think someone you know could be depressed, encour-age him to seek help. If he is feeling low and unable to think clearly, you may need to offer to take him to see his health care provider, a behavioral health specialist, or a social service agency in your community. Encourage him to join a support group to meet other people who are learning to cope with chronic dis-eases so he feels less alone.

Symptoms of Depression

- changes in appetite
- unexplained crying
- feeling restless
- feelings of hopelessness and sadness
- feelings of worthlessness
- headaches
- loss of energy
- loss of interest in favorite activities
- difficulty sleeping
- trouble remembering things
- trouble thinking clearly or making decisions
- thoughts of death or suicide

Q. Because I'm scared my girlfriend could have an insulin reaction, I worry about her and feel like I'm nagging her to check her glucose level all the time. I think I'm getting on her nerves. What should I do?

A. If you think you're nagging her, you probably are. It's natural to worry a little about lows. However, if you're worrying a lot, you need to identify what is causing the worry and making it into a worry-habit. If it continues, it could become destructive to your relationship.

The next time you are feeling anxious about a low happening, try to identify what it is that scares you the most about what could happen. Discuss this with your girlfriend. Ask her to help you understand how she feels when she has a low and how she treats it. Find out if she can usually tell when she is having a low and is able to treat it on her own. If you're worrying about hypoglycemia when she is able to catch and promptly treat lows (hypoglycemia) on her own, you are probably worrying too much. To resolve your worry, you need to learn to trust her and have confidence that she is able to take care of herself on her own. You also need to learn how and if she wants you to help her with her diabetes. Otherwise, she may find your constant worrying or hovering over her irritating.

How can I help? If you think you're catching low blood glucose levels before someone with diabetes is, try conducting a little experiment. The next five times she tests her glucose level, try to guess her glucose reading (number) before her glucose meter gives a result. Have her guess, too. Then make a pact that she'll test her blood glucose level the next couple of times you think she's low, but she doesn't. See who's right more often. You may be surprised at what you learn.

Q. My mother lives alone in her own house. Because I don't live near her, I worry about her becoming hypoglycemic and not being able to treat herself. How can I help her, and ease my worry?

A. People with diabetes who take insulin and live or spend much of their time alone should always take precautions to prevent hypoglycemia. If they have a low when they're alone and are unable to treat themselves, it could be a while before someone realizes they need assistance. For this reason, doctors encourage those people with diabetes who live alone to have a plan so that every day they check in with someone to ensure they're feeling all right. A plan may be to have a roommate or establish a safety check-in system. A safety check-in system consists of creating a plan where every day they either check in with someone or someone checks in on them. This way, if they have a low and need help, it will be close at hand.

You can help your mother by helping her create a check-in system if she hasn't done so already. Besides assuring you of her safety, check-in systems are a great way for older adults who live alone to retain their independence and remain socially connected to people. To create a check-in system, you need to do two things. First, have her identify one to three people she either talks to or sees each day. They could be friends, neighbors, coworkers, or relatives that she talks with. Have her ask them if they would be willing to be a "checker" for you. If they are, they agree to alert you or someone else if they notice that your mother needs help. By utilizing her existing friendships, she can even create a buddy system where she checks up on someone while they in turn check up on her. Second, create an emergency calling tree and have her share it with her appointed "checkers," so they know who to contact in case she needs help. The underlying point of the check-in system is to establish a plan where someone will take quick action in your absence, to get your mother assistance. Here's how to set it up.

Long-Distance Caring through Check-In Systems

Create an Emergency Calling Tree (Notification) Plan. Identify with your mother ahead of time the names and phone numbers of the following:

- her doctor
- her pharmacy
- her dentist
- the office where she works
- which hospital she wants to be taken to
- her health insurance information
- names of people who could help her in case of an emergency

Create Communication Checkpoints. Identify with your mother who will be a "checker" for you and her.

- Use the telephone or Internet to talk on a regular basis.
- If your mother has a friend or family member whom she talks with every day, ask that person to call her if they haven't heard from her by a certain time. If she doesn't respond, they should call you or initiate the emergency plan you've set up.

- If your mother works, have her ask either a co-worker or her manager to call her to verify she's okay if she fails to report for work. If she doesn't answer her phone, they know to initiate the emergency plan you've set up.

- If she regularly eats at a senior meal site and fails to show up, have her friends at the site check up on her—she can do the same for them if they don't show up.

- If your mother lives in a senior citizen complex, ask the manager or case manager (if there is one) if there are processes or systems in place at the complex so that people can check up on each other for health and safety.

- If your mother has a home security system, she can check to see if the system can include initiating the emergency plan if she doesn't turn off her system by a certain time each day.

- See if your mother can enroll in a "first alert" program, where if she has health problems she can alert emergency health personnel to check on her at the push of a button.

- If both you and your mother have Internet access, send each other quick "good morning" messages to start your day. If you don't hear from her by a certain time, you'll know to call her and see if she's okay.

- Contact your mother's health care provider to learn what social service programs exist in her area that can help maintain your mother's independent living style as long as possible.

Create Visual Checkpoints

- If a neighbor doesn't see your mother pick up her morning paper that's delivered in front of her door by 9:00 A.M., ask the neighbor to call or check to see if she's feeling okay.

- If a neighbor doesn't see your mother open up a certain window curtain by 9:00 A.M., ask the neighbor to call or check to see if she is feeling okay. You can also ask the neighbor to call you if something looks out of the norm.

Q. My husband has had diabetes for years, and lately he's been having a problem with impotence. Can diabetes cause sexual problems? I really miss being intimate with my husband and hate to think this is how it's going to be for the rest of our lives.

A. While sexual dysfunction can be caused by physical and psychological factors—for example, obesity, high blood pressure, anxiety, guilt, stress, and depression—it can also be caused by diabetes in both men and women. It's estimated that 30 percent of men and 35 percent of women with well-controlled diabetes suffer sexual problems due to the disease. If they have diabetes complications that have already set in, the rates for dysfunction increase to 40 to 50 percent in women and over 50 percent in men.

In men, the most common sexual dysfunction experienced is impotence. It develops gradually over time as a result of nerve damage (peripheral neuropathy) and/or a reduction in blood flow to the penis. In women, the most common problems reported are vaginal dryness, a loss of feeling in the genital area, and painful intercourse due to frequent urinary tract infections. When blood glucose levels are high, women and men report a decreased sex drive that resolves once glucose levels are normalized.

So what does this mean for you as a spouse or significant other? It means that it's important that you talk openly with each other about your fears and concerns so that together you can cope with the problem. Because diabetes is only one cause of sexual dysfunction, you may find it helpful to meet with his doctor or urologist to review the situation. While you both may feel uncomfortable talking with a doctor about this, there are a number of tests and treatments that men and women can use to improve sexual function. You may also find it helpful to meet with a counselor to explore and learn new ways to share intimacy that are pleasurable.

Q. Because I am so afraid my husband will have a low while he's sleeping, I stay up some nights watching him sleep to make sure he's okay. How can I get over this fear so that I can get a good night's sleep?

A. If you fear your husband will have a nighttime low, you need to assess whether your fear is justifiable or based on feeling overly protective. If your fear is based on the fact that he has been having frequent lows, your fear is justified and warrants discussing the lows with his health care provider. With the help of his doctor, together you can create a plan to prevent lows and let you both get a good night's rest. This may be achieved by adjusting his medications (or insulin) and having him eat a larger snack before going to bed. He may also need to regularly test his blood glucose level before going to sleep and occasionally during the middle of the night.

If your fear, however, is based on a single hypoglycemic episode that occurred in the past that made you feel helpless, your fear may be causing you to overreact. While you want to protect your husband, you can't sacrifice your health by not sleeping. If you haven't discussed your fears with your husband, you need to do so. Work together to help you build confidence and trust that he'll be okay at night. To do this, find out if he wakes up on his own when he has a low. Review the symptoms he has when he has a nighttime low. Establish a plan for how you can help him treat a low at night.

If you still find yourself worrying at night, then take ten slow, deep breaths and remind yourself that watching him sleep won't keep his glucose level up, only good diabetes management can do that. If he's taking good care of himself and hasn't had a low for months or years, rest confident that he's okay. However, if your fear remains, consider talking with a diabetes educator, counselor, or someone who can help support you and teach you additional ways to cope with your emotions.

Q. When I accompany my spouse to his doctor's appointment for diabetes, I know he sometimes lies about what he

eats and his self-care routine. I worry that if he's not truth-ful to his doctor, he won't get the diabetes care he needs. Should I speak up and tell his doctor he's lying?

A. Because you're concerned about your husband's health, it's natural to worry in a situation like this. As you know, your hus-band is only hurting himself by not being honest with himself and his doctor. Although he probably knows it's important that his doctor know how he is caring or not caring for himself, by not sharing this information, he loses out on opportunities to better care for his condition. However, like a child fears telling a teacher he didn't complete his homework, your husband may fear telling his doctor the truth.

Before your husband's next medical appointment, talk with him about what he is going to say. Help him make a list of ques-tions to ask his doctor or diabetes educator that he would like answered or addressed. Let him know, while you talk, that you know he hasn't always told the truth about his diet or self-care in the past. Remind him that his doctor will be able to tell when he's not taking the best care of his diabetes through the results of his blood tests (especially the glycated hemoglobin test and cho-lesterol level), so he shouldn't think he's fooling anyone by not telling the truth. And if there is something about his diet or self-care program that he doesn't like or finds too difficult to do, by talking with his doctor he may be able to learn ways to better cope with his disease and feel less controlled by it.

At your husband's next appointment, watch to see if he is more open about his diabetes care with his doctor. If he is, acknowledge his efforts and let him know how proud you are of him for doing so. If he doesn't tell the truth, ask your husband for permission to call his doctor to talk about his diabetes so you can learn how you can help him with his diet and self-care.

CHAPTER 8

Promoting Healthy Habits at Home

I FEEL LIKE I AM ALWAYS NAGGING MY DAD TO TAKE CARE OF HIMSELF
AND HIS DIABETES. HOW CAN I GET HIM TO CHANGE?

Have you ever wished you could get someone to change a habit or behavior that bothers you? Maybe you've wished one of your friends would quit smoking or that your spouse would stop working long hours and spend more time with the family. Maybe you wished something as simple as having a roommate clean up his dirty dishes after he gets done cooking instead of leaving them in the sink to get smelly. If you tried nagging someone to change, you know it doesn't work. That's because you can't make or force people to change, they have to see a reason to want to change themselves.

So how can you get someone to change or do something they don't want to? The answer is, you need to start with yourself. While that's probably not the answer you wanted or expected to hear, it is where you really need to start. You need to learn what motivates people to want to change and be successful at doing so. You need to know how to assess how ready or not to make changes someone is, and learn ways to persuade them to contemplate the idea of changing. Also, you'll need to learn what helps or hinders someone's efforts to change so that you don't unintentionally create roadblocks for them as they try to change.

The bottom line is this: changing habits doesn't happen overnight or by magic. If you know someone who has stopped smoking cigarettes, you know it can take several attempts before he is finally able to successfully quit. Breaking a bad habit takes time. Sometimes it can take weeks, months, or often years of hard work and persistence before it becomes a new habit. While this isn't meant to discourage you, it's to emphasize that when someone starts to change a habit, it may be a bumpy ride that takes longer than you expect.

This chapter will help you learn how change occurs and how to plan for it. You'll learn how to assess your—or someone else's—readiness to change a behavior that is unhealthy. You will also learn tips on how to encourage and support someone trying to change or break an unhealthy habit. So let's begin by reviewing how a person's family can both negatively and positively affect someone's health.

Q. I've always thought that diabetes was my husband's problem, not mine. Can our family's habits really have an effect on how well he controls his diabetes?

A. Yes. There is considerable data that indicate that the environment a person with diabetes lives in can influence how well he is able to cope with and manage his disease. A person's family can play a powerful role promoting and supporting the person with diabetes to care for his health.

People with diabetes and their spouses who report high marital satisfaction, good family organization skills, and low family stress report that they often have an easier time adopting and maintaining healthy lifestyle behaviors. On the flip side, high levels of stress, parenting concerns, financial problems, work problems, extended families, family conflicts, and low spouse involvement can negatively impact on a person's ability to positively manage diabetes.

Q. What does promoting health mean?

A. When people are faced with diabetes, illness, or physical or emotional impairments, they are forced to stop and reflect on their health and they way they live their lives. To have good health means to either be free from disease or in good physical and mental condition. But when someone has diabetes, being healthy requires taking action to control the disease. This means that she needs to act or behave in ways that reduce her risk for further disease, health complications, or premature death.

When you want someone to live in such a way that she remains healthy, you are encouraging or promoting health. For example, if you want a loved one to stop smoking cigarettes, you may be motivated by a desire to prevent lung cancer. However, simply wanting her to quit isn't going to get her to stop smoking. To help her be successful at stopping to smoke, you need to make sure she has an environment—at home, work, and school—that supports change. If everyone she associates with smokes or she smokes to cope with stress, it will be hard for her to successfully change unless she learns new ways to cope with stress and can restructure her environment so that triggers for smoking are reduced.

> **How can I help?**
> Create environments—at home or work—that encourage and support the people you love to live healthy lifestyles.

Q. My husband knows he should eat healthier foods, but he doesn't want to change. He says he doesn't want to give up his few remaining vices in the world—cookies, chips, and watching television all weekend—since he doesn't smoke or drink alcohol. I get so mad that he doesn't take better care of his health and doesn't stop doing things that he knows are bad for his diabetes. What can I do?

A. It's a simple fact that you can't make someone do something he doesn't want to do. He is responsible for the actions he takes, and only he can change his actions if he wants to.

Sometimes when people have diabetes, they can feel as if their condition controls their life. This is because treating diabetes often requires them to form many new habits all at once—

eating less sweets, exercising more, managing stress, testing blood glucose levels, taking medication. This can make them feel as if the diabetes treatment is dictating their life. If they have had little diabetes education or are still struggling to accept the fact that they have diabetes, they may feel at a loss as to how they can control their life. So they may decide to eat certain foods—like a cookie between meals—to rebel, even though they know the affect it will have on their blood glucose level. They do it because they can, and they decide they want to. However, the control they feel is an illusion, because they can't control the consequences of what happens in their body after they eat the cookie. Instead of working with their body to control the glucose, they're working against it, which increases their risk for health complications later on in life.

As humans, we have the ability to choose how to react in different situations. Stephen Covey in his book *Seven Habits of Highly Effective People* suggests that our attitudes and behaviors are influenced by how we view life and the personal values we believe in. When we make decisions, we can do so reactively or proactively. Reactive decisions are like knee-jerk responses to situations that happen around us. Decisions made or actions taken are reactions to how we feel in particular situations and circumstances. For example, if the weather is gloomy outside, we may react by feeling sad or uninspired. Or if there is a fire, we quickly react by trying to put it out.

Unfortunately, if diabetes care decisions are made only in a reactive way, it can cause him to feel controlled by his disease—always trying to chase after a blood glucose level. If his level is high, he may eat food intentionally to try to bring the number down. However, if he eats so little food that he remains hungry—he may feel unsatisfied and overeat later on.

On the other hand, if a person makes decisions based on internal beliefs combined with knowledge, he can make proactive decisions. Proactive people tend to see opportunities where others only see barriers. They don't let a little bad weather ruin their day, because they believe that regardless of what the weather is like, they can have a good day. Through proactive decisions, people can feel more in control of their destiny and diabetes because they make decisions by planning ahead to solve and prevent problems. A person with high blood glucose levels would reflect back to earlier in the day to determine what may have caused it. He may decide to follow a more intensive diabetes treatment program so he can understand how to better control his diabetes through diet, exercise, and medications.

Is your spouse reactive or proactive? Complete the activity below to find out.

Activity: Identifying Reactive vs. Proactive People

Directions: As you listen to people talk about their diabetes, see if you hear them saying any of the following phrases. If you spot reactive thinking, help them become more proactive so they feel more in control of their condition.

Reactive Thinking	Proactive Thinking
I can't change.	I can choose.
They won't let me.	What are my options?
She won't allow me to . . .	I prefer to . . .
If only I could . . .	I can change . . .
I have to . . .	I want to . . .

What can be hard for a friend or family member of a reactive thinker is that we may want them to change a behavior because we believe a different way would be best for him. But that's our belief, not his. Until he believes change is needed, he won't change. Nagging or trying to force him to change will only make him more resistant to the idea.

So what can you do? To help someone change health habits, it's important to first stop and take a few minutes to understand why he does what he does. Does he feel in control of his disease? Does he want to change any habits? Does he see any value in changing his behavior? Does he have the skills or knowledge to know how to change? If he gives up an old behavior (or favorite food), does he have a new one he can use instead? Is he scared to change? After you understand his point of view, you can help increase his awareness of the conse-quences of his actions and the benefits he will receive if he changes his choices and habits.

> *How can I help? Remember, any change he makes is better than no change at all. Recognize all efforts people make to change, especially the small ones. It's the first small steps they take that are most important in building their confidence that they can succeed.*

Q. What motivates a person to want to lead a healthy lifestyle and care for her diabetes?

A. Because each person with diabetes is different, there are countless reasons that can influence someone's decision on how she cares for her diabetes. Studies interviewing people with diabetes have found that some of the most common demotivators include: how much they know about diabetes (many lack knowledge), poor access to health care, lack of time, financial concerns, cultural values, poor family support, and poor coping skills. Those who find it hard to follow their diet report being influenced by how their family prefers to eat and the perception that healthy food doesn't taste good. Barriers to being physically active include physical discomfort, fear of hypoglycemia, lack of time and proper equipment, and lack of support from family members.

Q. I feel like I'm always telling my grandmother to quit eating foods that are bad for her. How can I get her to change and eat what she's supposed to without nagging?

A. Change is not an event that usually happens overnight, it's a process that happens over time. According to James Prochaska, John Norcross, and Carlo DiClemente in their book *Changing for Good*, when people change a lifestyle habit, they go through five predictable stages before they are successful. Each stage takes place over a period of time (months to, sometimes, years). People may go forward and backward as they go through the stages, but each step forward takes them closer to long-term success.

By understanding which stage a person is at for certain habits, you can learn ways to help her think about changing a habit, take steps to change, and eventually maintain the new habit she forms.

The five stages in this model are *precontemplation, contemplation, preparation, action,* and *maintenance.* To help you understand more about each stage, imagine how you would respond to the situation below.

Imagine that you love to start your morning off drinking a couple of mugs of hot black coffee. You've done this for over twenty years and feel the need to drink coffee to help get you going in the morning. However, your doctor just advised you to quit drinking coffee due to your health. What do you do?

A. Keep drinking the coffee, as you don't see what's so bad about it.

B. Keep drinking the coffee, but think about maybe cutting back or stopping sometime over the next year.

C. Agree to stop drinking coffee over the next couple of weeks.

D. You stopped drinking coffee last week and don't think staying away from it will be a problem for you as you've started drinking decaffeinated tea already.

E. You already anticipated he would advise giving up coffee, so you gave it up a couple of months ago.

Which response did you pick?

If you picked A, your response is consistent with being in the precontemplation stage. Precontemplators, when asked to change a habit or behavior, see no reason to change and have no intention of doing so. They don't see their behavior as a problem, and when the topic comes up they prefer to change the subject.

If you picked B, your response is consistent with being in the contemplation stage. Contemplators agree that there is probably a need for them to change their behavior sometime over the next six months, but aren't prepared to start right away. They aren't sure if the benefits of changing their behavior are worth the risk of giving up something they enjoy doing. They prefer to think about the situation for a while before taking any action.

If you picked C, your response is consistent with the preparation stage. People in this stage agree that there is a need to change their behavior and are ready to start. At first they may start by making some small changes in their behavior to see how it goes. They may also seek ways to learn how to start making changes.

If you picked D, your response is consistent with the action stage. People in the action stage have taken the first big step and have actually changed their behavior. They are enthusiastic about what they've started to do, but are at risk for relapse (falling back into their old behavior) over the next six months.

If you picked E, your response is consistent with the maintenance stage. People in this stage have held on to their new behavior for at least six months and are finding that the new habit is part of their new routine. They don't think about doing the old habit anymore and are finding that they don't even miss it. They're positive about the change they've made and plan to keep it up.

> *How can I help?*
> *Be patient and remember that change takes time because it's a process, not an event.*

Q. How can I tell which stage someone is in for changing a habit?

A. There are common characteristics and expressions that people use that can help you identify which stage they are in. These are listed on pages 228–230. It's easy to assess how ready someone is to change a habit or behavior by following these three steps.

Steps to Assess Someone's Stage of Change

1. *Communicate your concern.* If you've noticed a troublesome behavior that someone has, let him know you're concerned and explain why. Because he may not be aware that his behavior is a problem or not feel concerned about it, be tactful and gentle as you point out your observation. Your goal is not to put him on the defensive and start an argument. For example, you could say, *"Honey, I've noticed you've been eating a lot of cookies lately. I'm concerned about what that could be doing to your diabetes control. What do you think?"*

2. *Listen to his response.* If he responds by becoming defensive, denying that a problem exists, blaming the behavior on something else, or telling you to mind your own business, he is most likely in the precontemplation stage. However, if he agrees with your observation that he has a problem resisting cookies, he is in the contemplation stage.

3. *Ask him if he is ready to change.* If he agrees that his behavior needs to be changed, ask him when he would be ready to start making a change. If he says he would like to think about it for a while, he's in the contemplation stage. If he would like to start right away, he is at the preparation stage. If he responds by telling you that he's already started trying to change, acknowledge his efforts and let him know that you agree he made a good decision. If he has been making the change for less than six months, he is in the action stage. However, if the change has lasted more than six months, he is in the maintenance stage.

How to Recognize What Stage Someone Is At		
Stage of Change	**Common Characteristics**	**Common Expressions They'll Use**
Precontemplation	Doesn't realize he has a problem	It's not my problem—it's yours!
	Sees no reason to change	I don't have to do that.
	Prefers to change the subject	I don't want to talk about it.
	Lacks knowledge of the subject	It's impossible for me to change.
	Shifts blame to something else	Quit nagging me. Pick on someone else.

Stage of Change	Common Characteristics	Common Expressions They'll Use
Contemplation	Acknowledges a problem exists, but isn't ready to change yet	I know I should, but . . .
	Considering the impact a change could have on his life	I'm not sure if changing is worth it . . .
	Open to talking about the problem behavior	I don't understand . . . tell me about it . . . please explain . . .
	Wishes an easy solution existed	Changing takes too much work . . . couldn't you just do it for me?
	Searching for the perfect time to start	I'll change when the time is right . . . maybe next year . . .
Preparation	Ready to start changing	Let's start . . . sign me up!
	Wants help getting started	What do I need to do?
	Wants an action plan	How and when can I start?
	Sees benefits to changing	If I start walking, I'll have more energy!
	Open to trying small changes	I'll try switching from 2% milk to skim milk.
Action	Actively changing an old habit into a new one	I used to drink regular soda, but now I'm only drinking diet!
	Change is noticeable to others	Oh, you noticed! Yes, I switched to . . . or started . . .
	Believes he can succeed	I was amazed to learn . . .
	Starting to change his environment in order to succeed	I cleaned out my cupboards and got rid of all the high-sodium condiments I had, and bought new spices.
	At risk for slipping back into old habits	I really wanted to eat some holiday candy, but I resisted it.
Maintenance	New habit is easy to do	I don't even think about it any more, I just do it . . .
	Has worked the new habit into his lifestyle	I'm very confident that I can . . . you know, I really enjoy walking outside in the mornings for exercise now because it gives me a chance to greet my neighbors!
	Plans ahead to prevent relapse	I planned ahead for this weekend when my children visit. I have lots of fruits and vegetables on hand for everyone to snack on.

continued

Stage of Change	Common Characteristics	Common Expressions They'll Use
Maintenance (continued)	Continues to modify his environment	I put away all the old candy dishes I used to have out.... We don't use them anymore, so it didn't make sense having them clutter up the counter ... I found a really pretty plant to put on the counter instead ... it's much prettier to look at!
	Reminds himself that he made the right decision	I feel good about my decision ... because I started walking for exercise, I have more energy to play with my grandchildren!

Source: Adapted with permission from "Stages of Change Counseling Grid," Center for Health Promotion, Health Partners, All Rights Reserved, 1999.

Q. How can I motivate someone to change once I have identified the stage she is in?

A. Once you know which stage of change a person is in, your attitude toward her will play a large role in your success in helping her to change. If you don't believe or think she can change, it will be hard to show enthusiasm for any efforts she makes. Don't demand that she change—inspire her to want to do it. Help her identify the benefits she'll receive if she changes. If you can make it worth her while, chances are that pretty soon she'll be asking how she can start changing.

If someone is in the precontemplation stage of change, you can't force her or demand that she change as she sees no reason to change. To help motivate her to start thinking about changing her habits, you'll want to try to understand why she is acting the way she is. Subtly help her become aware that a habit she has is problematic and that she has options she could take to change. Encourage her just to think about the effect her habit has on her health and those around her.

After someone becomes aware that she has a problem and acknowledges it, she will start to think about it and what she could do to change. However, to help her make any decisions, she needs to first understand all the facts. Is she aware of how her actions affect her blood glucose level? Is she aware of the benefits she will have if she changes? If she is grappling with anger and fear about diabetes or hasn't come to accept her disease, she could stay in this thinking stage for months to years if she has more internal reasons for not changing than benefits for changing.

To help motivate her to change, listen to her concerns. Don't be judgmental or preach. By showing empathy, you can help her cope emotionally with her disease. Address the reasons and concerns she has for not wanting to change and, hard as it may be at first, accept the decisions she makes without feeling guilty or casting blame. Over time, if she can start to learn how her behavior affects her health, she can start to see the benefits of change. You'll need to help her identify the barriers she has to changing and provide options for getting around them.

Once she decides she wants to change, she has reached the stage where she's ready, willing, and motivated to start. You'll want to take advantage of her enthusiasm to help her come up with a plan to start changing. When she's at this stage, it's the motivational moment you've been waiting for. It's similar to someone getting her ears pierced for the first time; once she is ready to do it, she wants to just do it and be done before she changes her mind.

When she is ready to start, it's important that you remind her that changing habits takes hard work. Set realistic goals and expectations with her as to what's possible to achieve. While she may want a major overhaul of her lifestyle habits (e.g., eat better, exercise more, lose weight, stop smoking, or reduce stress at work), help her to pick one habit to start with. Encourage one change at a time. Encourage her to learn the new skills she'll need to successfully change the habit she picks. This may consist of reading books, enrolling in classes, or talking to an educator or counselor who can teach her those skills. The more options she has to choose from, the more in control of her decision to change she will feel.

After she's started making changes, she'll need your support and encouragement as she enters the action and maintenance stages. This is where it's extremely important that you help her create an environment at home, work, and school where she can successfully maintain the changes she's started. For example, if she wants to eat fewer high-fat or sugary foods, try not to bake cookies or keep candy in the house that is tempting to eat. If she wants to become more active, offer to join her for a walk together, do a recreational sport you both enjoy, or take up a hobby. At the same time, don't let her forget what she's accomplished and be supportive when she has occasional lapses into her old habits. Lapses happen and should be expected. Here are some suggestions for do's and don'ts to remember when trying to encourage someone to change a behavior.

Do's (Remember to):

- listen to what she says and feels
- praise her accomplishments in front of others
- provide her with correct health information, as needed
- review the benefits she has from changing a habit
- identify barriers to changing a habit

Don'ts (Try Not to):

- be too picky or judgmental, or critical
- nag, preach, or demand she change
- forget to notice her efforts, no matter how small
- scold her when she slips into old habits

How can I help? Encourage change by giving people choices. Research suggests that people are more likely to be successful at changing habits when they have two or three choices to decide between.

Q. What can I do if my husband doesn't want to test his blood glucose level? (The doctor can't even get him to do it!)

A. If you've discussed with your husband the concerns you have about his behavior and he decides he doesn't want to change, that's a decision he has made. Although you may disagree, you need to accept that he's made a decision. No amount of coaxing or pushing is going to get him to change until he's ready.

Instead of begging or pestering him to change, what you need to do is talk with him and listen to determine the reasons why he doesn't want to test his blood glucose level. Try to understand how he made his decision (what his goals, values, and beliefs are) and then acknowledge his feelings. Let him know that while you don't agree with his decision, you still love him. This way he will know he's responsible for his decision and that you're not going to demand he do something he doesn't believe in doing. But at the same time, continue to let him know that you care about him and his health. Enlist the aid of his family and friends to let him know they care about him, but also let him know the effect of his decision upon their lives and relationships with him. Don't forget to ask him every now and then if he wants to reconsider and change his mind.

At this stage, it may be hard for you to be patient and not demand that he change. If you nag or pester him, he may rebel and not listen to your reasons for changing. He needs to believe he has the choice to think about changing his behavior and has options he can pick from.

How can I help? Once someone has made an effort to form a new habit, don't forget that he has changed and hold his former habit against him. For example, if he used to run late for family gatherings but has changed over the past year and now makes an effort to be prompt, don't tease or call him "last one to show up" anymore, as that is no longer true. It demotivates the person from continuing his new habit because of your attitude toward him.

Q. Why can't my sister stick to her diet? It seems like she does well for a while, and then she falls off the wagon and slips into her old habits.

A. You need to understand and appreciate that changing habits takes time and a lot of hard work. When someone starts to make lifestyle changes, she is automatically at risk for falling back into her old habits when new situations arise or life gets a little stressful. For example, she can have the best plan to keep eating a low-fat diet, but when holiday season rolls around she may lapse into old eating habits when faced with a lot of old favorite foods that are high in fat and calories.

Lapses are normal and should be expected. When lapses are treated as a simple "oops" without a lot of fuss being made or having the event blown up out of proportion, chances are your sister will get back to her new eating habits as soon as the temptation of the holiday food is removed. But by planning ahead, you and your sister can proactively work to identify the times when it gets hard for her to stay on her diet and strategize ways to prevent lapses from happening. Maybe next year during the holidays you could try modifying some of her favorite old recipes to make them healthier, or help her learn how to fit a small slice of a favorite food into her meal plan without compromising her diabetes control. Better yet, decide if you need to have all the sweets around and offer healthier snacks instead.

> **How can I help?**
> Help create a supportive environment for people where failure isn't fatal and they are encouraged to learn from their mistakes and try again.

Q. If someone cheats on his diet every now and then, that's okay, isn't it?

A. The word "cheat" means to deliberately deceive or trick. When someone cheats on his diet, the only person he's hurting is himself. Sure, he can get away with eating something occasionally that he shouldn't. The risk is that if he gets away with it today, will he try it again tomorrow and the next day? Will he be ready to pay the price for having poor blood glucose control later in life if he develops health problems from his diabetes? Are you ready to accept responsibility for his health if you encourage him to cheat?

Ask yourself, "Do I ever encourage him to not follow his diet? Do I ever urge him to have just a small piece of something when he doesn't feel like eating? Have I ever told him to 'just go ahead and have some' when he was hesitating?" If you have, you've helped and encouraged him to cheat. When you do this, then you share some of the responsibility for his health. But when he decides to cheat on his own, it's his responsibility to understand the consequences of his actions.

If you want to help him stay healthy, think of the diet as a prescribed treatment he is required to take, just like medication. Ask yourself, Would I encourage him to cheat on taking his medication? Would I say, "Oh, you can skip taking your medication today—nobody will know?" No. That isn't something anyone would do, as we all know that people take medication to stay healthy. Well, the diet is the same way. People aren't prescribed a diet as a punishment—diets are a treatment method. His diet is a meal plan that is tailored to meet his special health needs and helps him control his diabetes.

> **How can I help?**
> Don't encourage your loved one to cheat on his diet by pushing food at him. It only makes it harder for him to follow his diet without disappointing you.

Sometimes we feel so bad when someone has diabetes that we try to make them feel better by offering treats that we enjoy. However, this puts them in a dilemma. People who don't snack on treats do not miss them. When you "push food" on them, it is hard for them to follow their diets, and instead of the food making them feel better, they may eat the food only to please you—not them.

Q. My husband and his parents all have type 2 diabetes. His parents are always telling me that I should be helping my husband eat better. However, they don't realize that I do try to help him with his diet, but he doesn't want to eat the food I make him. They nag me and I nag him, but it isn't getting anywhere except giving me a headache. What can I do?

A. It sounds like you're caught in a cycle that is making you feel trapped—like being stuck in an elevator caught between floors. Your body's reaction to the situation is that you're becoming stressed and angry. While you realize the problem is that your husband doesn't want to eat healthy, the strategy both his parents and you have been using, nagging, isn't working. It's only building resentment.

You need to be honest with your in-laws and let them know that you agree with their concern for their son. Let them know that you've been preparing healthy meals for him and your family and encouraging him to eat healthfully. However, while you appreciate their concern, ask that they express their concern directly to your husband instead, as he is the one who needs to hear it. While they may have learned to cope well with their diabetes, your husband hasn't. By working together, you can help increase your husband's awareness that his eating habits are affecting others. Help him understand how the benefits of changing his habits outweigh his risk in continuing them. But remember, it's his choice to make whether he follows his diet or not. Don't take the blame for his decision.

CHAPTER 9

Building Positive Relationships

MY BOYFRIEND DOESN'T LIKE TO TALK ABOUT HIS DIABETES.
WHEN I TRY TO GET HIM TO TALK ABOUT IT, HE JUST SHRUGS HIS
SHOULDERS AND SAYS HE'S OK AND NOT TO WORRY ABOUT HIM, BUT I DO.
HOW CAN I GET HIM TO UNDERSTAND I CARE AND WANT TO HELP?

Have you ever wished you could get to know someone better? Maybe it was a coworker, a friend, or a relative. By expressing interest in knowing someone, you're building a relationship or friendship with them.

Friendships are wonderful things that have magical qualities. Friends can brighten a gloomy day by just the sharing of a smile or a hug. In times of trouble, a friendly word of encouragement or advice can encourage you to try a little harder and feel a little less alone. Friends also remember to celebrate and share with each other the joys and accomplishments of life.

However, for friendships to grow and flourish between people, they require an investment of time and energy to make the relationship work. They require communication, genuine concern, and caring for their each other's well-being.

When someone has diabetes, the disease can add another dimension to a relationship. This doesn't mean to imply that the dimension is either good or bad; it simply recognizes the fact that diabetes is a part of who he is and requires his attention. As you build a relationship with someone who has diabetes, you can't ignore the fact that he needs to follow a certain meal schedule or take certain self-care to keep his blood glucose level under control.

To some people, diabetes can feel like a third person in your relationship. When meals and events run on schedule, diabetes acts like a "silent partner," and you may even forget that a person has it. However, if you become lax and get off schedule, it doesn't remain silent—instead, it acts up, forcing everyone to pay attention to it. If you have ever referred to someone's diabetes as, "because of his diabetes, we have to . . . ," you've already acknowledged that diabetes plays a role in your relationship.

This chapter will discuss some of the ingredients that make up positive relationships and friendships. You will learn ways you can help someone with diabetes by communicating openly and more effectively. The chapter will also give you ideas on how to build a supportive environment that encourages the person you know with diabetes to care for himself.

Q. What makes up a positive, supportive relationship?

A. If you were to name one or two people in your life who are important to you, who would they be? Would it be a parent or spouse, a family member, or a friend? Whoever you picked, you identified her as being important to you because you felt a connection with that person. That connection can best be described as a relationship.

Positive relationships are when two or more people form a bond or attachment between them that is built on feelings of trust, concern, honesty, and respect. Friendships can develop from relationships when feelings of mutual affection and common interests exist and people enjoy spending time being together. Good friends are those people you are glad to see regardless of what they look like, what time of day it is, or even what events may transpire to bring you together. When they call at midnight to say they have car trouble, you automatically ask where they are and how you can help. Because you care about each other, you want to help each other.

Q. My friend Janelle has diabetes. How can I help her with it?

A. Only your friend can tell you how you can help her cope with her diabetes. Therefore, start by asking her if she minds talking to you about her disease. If she doesn't, find out what is hard about having diabetes and get her ideas on how you can be supportive. In the process, you will learn how you can help and build a stronger friendship between the two of you. You will also officially become a "helper." Helpers are people who assist other people to understand or cope with a problem and can be either professional or informal helpers. Professional helpers are those people who are specially trained to counsel and help others (such as doctors, social workers, therapists, and teachers). You, on the other hand, will become an informal helper—a friend who reaches out to help in an honest and caring way.

To become an informal helper to someone involves three things. First, you need to understand what diabetes is (which you do from reading this book). Second, you need to be aware of your own personal health beliefs and habits. Once you recognize what your own values and opinions are about health and life, you will be able to better assess whether your actions are different or the same as that of the person you're trying to help. This is important because as a helper, you'll need to keep your opinions and beliefs to yourself, so you don't impose your values on her. Third, you need to have good listening skills so you can effectively communicate with the person you want to help. Good helpers are active listeners and give

> **How can I help?**
> *If you're not sure how to help someone with her diabetes, don't be shy—ask!*

constructive feedback. They don't preach or force someone to make decisions.

How can you tell if you have good self-awareness and communication skills? Find out by taking the following quiz.

Quiz: How Helpful Am I?

Directions: Think about the times you have spent with your friend or family member who has diabetes. Below are statements that relate to healthy eating, exercise, communication, and helper habits. For each statement, circle the number next to the response that best describes how often you would agree with the statement. Be as honest and accurate as you can. (*Note:* For consistency, the person with diabetes will be referred to as *he* or *him*.)

Eating Habits

1. **Eating meals together is difficult because he doesn't like the same foods I do.**

   ⑤ Strongly Agree   ④ Somewhat Agree   ③ Neutral
   ② Slightly Disagree   ① Disagree

2. **I feel impatient or embarrassed when he stops to test his blood glucose level before eating.**

   ⑤ Strongly Agree   ④ Somewhat Agree   ③ Neutral
   ② Slightly Disagree   ① Disagree

3. **To show him I love him, I like to bake him special meals and desserts.**

   ⑤ Strongly Agree   ④ Somewhat Agree   ③ Neutral
   ② Slightly Disagree   ① Disagree

4. **I often encourage him to cheat on his diet.**

   ⑤ Strongly Agree   ④ Somewhat Agree   ③ Neutral
   ② Slightly Disagree   ① Disagree

5. **I eat sweets or high-fat snack foods in front of him.**

   ⑤ Strongly Agree   ④ Somewhat Agree   ③ Neutral
   ② Slightly Disagree   ① Disagree

6. **I feel hurt when he doesn't eat large portions of the food I cook specially, just for him.**

   ⑤ Strongly Agree   ④ Somewhat Agree   ③ Neutral
   ② Slightly Disagree   ① Disagree

7. I watch what he eats and always let him know when I catch him cheating.

⑤ Strongly Agree   ④ Somewhat Agree   ③ Neutral
② Slightly Disagree   ① Disagree

Exercise Habits

8. I find excuses for us not to exercise or be physically active.

⑤ Strongly Agree   ④ Somewhat Agree   ③ Neutral
② Slightly Disagree   ① Disagree

9. I believe weekends and vacations are meant for sleeping late and watching television.

⑤ Strongly Agree   ④ Somewhat Agree   ③ Neutral
② Slightly Disagree   ① Disagree

10. We do not go out walking or exercise together.

⑤ Strongly Agree   ④ Somewhat Agree   ③ Neutral
② Slightly Disagree   ① Disagree

11. We always use escalators or elevators instead of stairs when we're at a mall shopping.

⑤ Strongly Agree   ④ Somewhat Agree   ③ Neutral
② Slightly Disagree   ① Disagree

12. I do not encourage him to do muscle conditioning exercises.

⑤ Strongly Agree   ④ Somewhat Agree   ③ Neutral
② Slightly Disagree   ① Disagree

13. We often delay or skip eating meals when we're busy doing things like working in the yard, golfing, or shopping.

⑤ Strongly Agree   ④ Somewhat Agree   ③ Neutral
② Slightly Disagree   ① Disagree

Communication Habits

14. I never interrupt him when he is talking.

⑤ Strongly Agree   ④ Somewhat Agree   ③ Neutral
② Slightly Disagree   ① Disagree

15. I always ask him to clarify or explain what he's saying when we talk.

⑤ Strongly Agree   ④ Somewhat Agree   ③ Neutral
② Slightly Disagree   ① Disagree

16. I always stop what I'm doing and focus my attention on him when he wants to talk.

⑤ Strongly Agree   ④ Somewhat Agree   ③ Neutral
② Slightly Disagree   ① Disagree

17. We shut off the radio or television when we want to have a serious conversation.

⑤ Strongly Agree   ④ Somewhat Agree   ③ Neutral
② Slightly Disagree   ① Disagree

18. I always praise him on how well he cares for his diabetes.

⑤ Strongly Agree   ④ Somewhat Agree   ③ Neutral
② Slightly Disagree   ① Disagree

19. We never disagree about how he cares for himself.

⑤ Strongly Agree   ④ Somewhat Agree   ③ Neutral
② Slightly Disagree   ① Disagree

Helper Habits

20. I always like to feel like I'm in control of a situation.

⑤ Strongly Agree   ④ Somewhat Agree   ③ Neutral
② Slightly Disagree   ① Disagree

21. When we have a discussion, I know I'm always right.

⑤ Strongly Agree   ④ Somewhat Agree   ③ Neutral
② Slightly Disagree   ① Disagree

22. **I like to give advice and solve other people's problems.**

⑤ Strongly Agree   ④ Somewhat Agree   ③ Neutral
② Slightly Disagree   ① Disagree

23. **I get upset when someone doesn't agree with me or do what I want to do.**

⑤ Strongly Agree   ④ Somewhat Agree   ③ Neutral
② Slightly Disagree   ① Disagree

24. **It's easy for me to compliment someone. I do it all the time.**

⑤ Strongly Agree   ④ Somewhat Agree   ③ Neutral
② Slightly Disagree   ① Disagree

25. **Talking about emotions and feelings (whether they're mine or someone else's) makes me feel uncomfortable.**

⑤ Strongly Agree   ④ Somewhat Agree   ③ Neutral
② Slightly Disagree   ① Disagree

Scoring: The number that you circled next to each of your responses represents the number of points assigned to that response. Within each of the four sections above, add up the number of points you circled to get a total score. Write your scores in the box below.

Total Eating Habits points	=	_____
Total Exercise Habits points	=	_____
Total Communication Habits points	=	_____
Total Helper Habits points	=	_____

Interpreting Your Scores

Eating Habits

7–15 points: Excellent	You're very sensitive to and supportive of your friend or family member's need to eat healthy. Keep up the good work!
16–25 points: Fair	You're sensitive to your friend or family member's diet needs, but sometimes encourage him to stray. Be more careful not to lead him into temptation.
26–35 points: Needs work	While you know he needs to be careful about what he eats, you're not always putting it into practice. Remember, actions speak louder than words. Support him by trying to deemphasize the role food plays in your relationship. Show him that you care by not encouraging him to overeat or munch on high-fat and high-calorie foods.

Exercise Habits

6–14 points: Awesome	Congratulations! You have healthy exercise habits and enjoy being physically active with your friend or family member who has diabetes. This is going to help both of you stay strong and healthy.
15–22 points: Fair	While you're aware of the benefits you can receive by being physically active, you're at risk for missing out on them yourself. Try to make more time for you and your friend or family member with diabetes to be active and healthy together for a lifetime.
23–30 points: Needs work	Careful, you're in danger of becoming an exercise saboteur. For both your health and theirs, it's important to remember the benefits you both can have from leading an active lifestyle—stay healthy, manage your weight,

look younger, feel more energetic, and reduce stress. Try not to discourage him or yourself from accumulating at least thirty minutes of physical activity each day. As you become more active, you may be amazed at how great you feel.

Communication Habits

6–14 points:
Full of potential

While your conversational skills are a little rusty, you have potential to be an effective communicator with a little practice. Watch your words and nonverbal actions a little more so that you don't miss out on what the other person is saying. Minimize distractions around you so that you can focus your attention on him when he talks, otherwise he may think you're not interested in him.

15–22 points:
Promising

Your conversational skills show a lot of promise. Practice polishing your listening skills as you let him do more of the talking when you're together. You may be surprised at what you hear and learn. Good luck!

23–30 points:
Very effective

Your communications skills are strong, and your strength lies in your ability to actively listen to what people are saying. Have you ever thought about being a professional helper?

Helper Habits

6–14 points:
Impressive

Wow! Your friends and family members must enjoy hanging out with you. Not only do you give them positive feedback, but you have a talent for being able to see two sides of an issue. Keep up the good work!

15–22 points:
Reasonable

You've got the ability to be a really good helper with practice. Try to take a neutral stance when you try to help someone so you don't come across as a know-it-all. To be an effective helper, practice your listening skills so that he has the final say in what concerns him, not you.

23–30 points:
Poor

While your helping skills may be poor at the moment, don't worry. When you care about someone and really want to help him succeed, you can become an effective helper if you start practicing the skills in the next section. Read on!

Q. How can I become an effective helper?

A. Effective helpers share common traits that enable them to assist others and make them feel good about themselves. They are respectful of the other's feelings, honest, sincere in their desire to help, and have a positive attitude toward life that rubs off on the person needing help. As someone who wants to help others, you may already have many of these traits and can build upon them as you practice your helping skills.

> *How can I help? Effective helpers don't try to change, fix, or solve problems for people. Their talent is in listening and offering options on how to change or solve a problem, but only when they're asked to.*

Helpers who are most effective at helping someone cope with a problem or health condition remember that their goal is to help, not take over and solve problems. Helpers are team players and encourage others to learn new skills and behaviors by helping them understand the consequences of their behavior. They ask probing, open-ended questions and carefully listen to discern what the problem is before identifying what options exist to possibly solve it. They also realize that since the problem isn't theirs, they need to draw the line at trying to change, fix, or solve it for the other person unless they are asked to. Only the person with the problem can decide when and how he wants to solve it.

When learning to become a helper, there are things you can do to inspire or hinder someone in successfully dealing with a problem. Below is a list of do's and don'ts to remember when trying to help someone. These are the skills to practice as you fine-tune your helping skills.

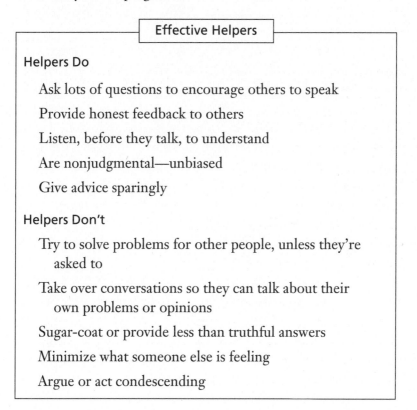

Effective Helpers

Helpers Do

Ask lots of questions to encourage others to speak

Provide honest feedback to others

Listen, before they talk, to understand

Are nonjudgmental—unbiased

Give advice sparingly

Helpers Don't

Try to solve problems for other people, unless they're asked to

Take over conversations so they can talk about their own problems or opinions

Sugar-coat or provide less than truthful answers

Minimize what someone else is feeling

Argue or act condescending

Q. My wife tells me I never listen to her. But that's because she likes to talk when my favorite television show is on. How can I become a better listener?

A. A good listener is an attentive listener who makes time to listen when someone talks—whether it's a spouse, child, or friend. Because it's difficult to listen to two things at once, if your body language and attention are focused on television rather than on the person talking, you are sending out signals that you don't feel the conversation is worth your time to listen to. This results in people feeling that they are unimportant to you.

Good listeners make a conscious effort to hear and understand what someone is trying to say. They listen by sight and by sound so they can hear not just what words are being said, but also how they are being said. Listening is a skill that people can learn and perfect with practice. While it comes naturally to some, others need to work at it.

Listening and communication skills naturally vary between women and men. According to John Gray in his book *Mars and Venus: Together Forever,* women are able to feel, think, and talk at the same time, whereas men prefer to think before talking. Often when wives complain to husbands that they don't listen, what they were trying to do is often share a concern with them and get confirmation that they were heard and understood. When they share the concern or problem, they are not always looking for an immediate solution. On the other hand, when men talk about a concern or problem, they assume that the point of the conversation is to find a solution that is quick and to the point.

Because men and women often communicate differently, some may have an easier time sharing their feelings than others. It's important to recognize this and let people know it's okay to talk about feelings when they are more comfortable doing so. Don't push—ask for permission instead so that they feel more open to sharing, if they want to.

The next time your wife, friend, or child wants to sit down and talk with you, follow these tips to become an attentive listener. If you do, you will find that listening can be a lot of fun, is enlightening, and can build a higher level of intimacy within a relationship.

Q. When I try to talk with my daughter before supper to find out how her blood glucose level is, she never wants to

---

Rules for Effective Listening

- If you're unable to talk when she wants to, schedule a time with her when you can give her your undivided attention to listen.

- Prepare to listen by minimizing noise and distractions around you, and giving the person talking your full attention.

- Show interest by making direct eye contact. (*Note*: In some cultures, avoiding eye contact is a sign of respect. If this is the case, show your respect by avoiding it.)

- Listen without interrupting or giving unwanted advice.

- Use facial expressions (smile) and nod while you listen, to communicate that you hear what she's saying.

- Repeat back (paraphrase) to her what you are hearing to make sure you understand correctly what she said and meant.

---

talk with me because we end up arguing. How can I be a better listener if she doesn't want to talk?

A. To facilitate effective communication, you need to create a supportive environment where your daughter feels open to talk. A supportive environment is one where she feels she can talk without being judged, preached to, or put on the spot. If your approach to starting the conversation puts her on the defensive, you'll end up arguing instead of listening.

Next time, try encouraging your daughter to talk by using the "ALT" approach to listening. The approach is easy to use and remember because it consists of just three simple steps—ask, listen, and think. Here's how it works. When you *ask* questions, use short, open-ended questions that begin with the word *who*, *where*, *what*, *how*, or *when*. Be careful asking *why* questions as they can often put someone automatically on the defensive.

This doesn't mean you can't ask a *why* question—just ask it tactfully. After each question, *listen* carefully to hear her answer. Don't argue or start a debate. Just let her talk. After she's done talking, take a moment to *think* about what she just said and *learn* what she's feeling. Then repeat the process again by asking her to clarify something she just said you'd like to understand more fully. By being patient and asking her to clarify her answers, you'll have a conversation going in no time that you both can feel good about. Here's how it works.

ALT Approach to Listening

Step 1.   *Ask* a question to start the conversation rolling.

Step 2.   *Listen* to what is said and acknowledge feelings. Don't interrupt, offer advice, or make hasty judgments.

Step 3.   *Think* about what is said. Do you fully understand what they meant?

Step 4.   Ask an open-ended question to have her clarify or explain further something she said—do this by asking a question starting with *who, where, what, how,* or *when* and phrasing your question to reflect back what she just said to show that you were listening but are seeking further understanding.

Step 5.   Repeat Steps 2 through 4 two more times, or as needed until you fully understand the problem at hand.

If you ever want to see a good example of the ALT approach in process, just watch how a toddler talks with a parent. Children are naturally curious and love to ask the question "why" as they explore the world around them. They will ask a parent a "why" question and then patiently listen for a response. For example, they may ask what color is the sky. When the parent answers "blue," they think about it for a while and then respond back with, "Why is the sky blue?" They continue to ask, listen, and think about it, using simple questions, until they receive an answer they can understand. (Sometimes, though, they ask more than 3 why questions.) Eventually, they end the conversation by saying "Oh, okay," and accept the conversation they just had without judgment and learn from it.

As we get older and learn more words, our conversations grow more complex than those that we have with toddlers. However, we can still use the simple ask-listen-learn concept to slow down and listen effectively to others. Below are two scenarios—one of an ineffective conversation and one using the ALT approach that is more effective. Notice how the tone and length of a conversation can change when you start by asking for information, acknowledging feelings, and listening for a complete answer.

Scenario 1: An Ineffective Conversation

You: How is your glucose level today?

Her: I don't know. I haven't tested.

You: You know better. You're supposed to test before supper. *(a hasty judgment that introduces blame into the conversation)*

Her: I don't like to. I don't have to do it every day. *(feeling defensive)*

You: The doctor said you should. *(condescending tone sounds like nagging)*

Her: Just drop it. It's my problem, not yours. *(feeling irritated; the conversation ends)*

Scenario 2: An Effective Conversation (Rephrased) Using the ALT Approach

You: How is your glucose level today?

Her: I don't know. I haven't tested yet.

You: Oh. *Why* not? *(first question to show simple curiosity and interest)*

Her: I don't know. It's such a pain. How would you like to have to do it every day? *(feeling defensive)*

You: Well, I probably wouldn't like it either. *What* is the worst thing about testing that makes it a pain? *(acknowledges her feeling and shows empathy; second question seeks further clarification)*

Her: Well, I can never get enough blood out of my finger when I poke it. So I end up having to poke it twice, which hurts. *(starting to feel listened to)*

You: Ow! I wouldn't like that either, *what* causes the first poke not to work? *(third question seeks further clarification)*

Her: I don't know. Maybe it's the calluses I have on my fingers from playing guitar.

You: Oh, I didn't know that. Gosh, having calluses must make it hard for everyone who has to poke their finger. I wonder if there is a different way to do it so you don't always have to poke twice? We could call your diabetes educator tomorrow and ask. *What* do you think? *(acknowledging the problem underlying why she doesn't like to test and offering a simple suggestion)*

Her: Anything would be worth a try. Thanks for listening and trying to understand.

How can I help? Having an effective conversation with someone requires that you focus your attention and really listen.

Q. I've been trying to help my husband with his diabetes for over ten years. I've read countless books and try to make sure he takes good care of himself. However, the

more I try to help him, the angrier at me he gets. What am I doing wrong?

A. Within all relationships, especially those where someone has diabetes or a chronic illness, it's sometimes natural to want to protect the person you care about. In trying to protect him, though, you may inadvertently treat him as if he is made of glass and could break if treated the wrong way. In an effort to understand his disease, you may become more motivated than he is to treat it by constantly encouraging him to change his behavior or act a different way. You become more of a professional coach to him than a helping spouse. How your husband is feeling could be similar to how a child feels whose parents want him to take more and more piano lessons because they are good for him—the child doesn't see the big picture, just the endless hours of practice sitting at a piano.

If this is the way your husband is feeling about his diabetes, your enthusiastic concern and ideas for his well-being are not what he wants to hear. Your concern and care for him has possibly gotten to a level of responsibility that is more than your husband wants. The more you do things for him, the more dependent it makes him on you, which can make him feel vulnerable. However, the more you do for him that seems unappreciated, the more resentful and angry you become. You may find it helpful to sit down and discuss with him your concerns and have him help you establish what responsibility, if any, he wants to share with you for his diabetes self-care.

While your intentions have been, and are admirable, he needs to retain as much independence as possible. He needs to be encouraged to care for himself, inasmuch as he is able to do, so that you don't become his caregiver if that's not what he needs or wants. While he may want to depend upon

How can I help? Build positive supporting relationships by encouraging each other to talk about the role each shares in the relationship and identifying who is responsible for doing what. This way, expectations are clearly defined and misunderstandings are avoided.

you for emotional support and help with some daily activities (e.g., cooking and shopping), he may not want to depend upon you for everything. Talk with him about this and define the role each of you plays within your relationship as husband and wife.

Once you redefine your roles and responsibilities toward each other, make sure you help him retain his independence. This is especially important in the event that someday you are not around to cook his meals or take care of day-to-day duties in your home. Would he know how to get along without you? Unfortunately, too often it's only after one spouse passes away that the other discovers he is left ill-prepared to care for himself because the spouse who left was the one who always did the cooking or paid the bills. Make sure both of you know how to cook, do laundry, and take care of finances. This way, you can help each other take care of each other in a healthy way.

Q. I get so frustrated trying to help my mother. I think she has either poor hearing or selective hearing, as whenever I go with her to her clinic appointments we argue afterward about what her doctor said. She says she heard him say one thing when I know he said something totally different. I'm tired of arguing with her. What can I do?

A. The answer is simple: get the doctor to put his directions in writing on a piece of paper so you've got his exact answer in black and white. Before you go to your mother's next doctor's appointment, contact him to explain your concern, that you suspect your mother may have poor or selective hearing. Enlist his help to check her hearing. Ask him to write down his instructions for her and ask her to repeat back the directions he gives to minimize misunderstandings.

In the process of having her hearing checked, you may discover that she needs a hearing aid. Changes in how well we hear are a part of the normal aging process. An estimated 75 percent of people over the age of seventy-five have hearing loss to the point that it causes difficulty with communication. The degree of hearing loss that people have is related to the volume and amount of noise they've been exposed to throughout their life. People with hearing loss often have problems hearing the middle and higher frequencies in speech. The letter sounds of F, T, D, S, SH, and Z become more difficult to hear and distinguish— speech seems less clear and hard to understand. If hearing loss isn't recognized and dealt with, it can be frustrating for everyone—you and her.

You can help people with hearing loss hear what is being said, if you follow these tips:

- When talking, try to lower your voice when you speak if you have a normally high voice.
- When talking, directly face her as you talk so she can read your lips.
- If you normally wear lipstick, wear a brighter shade if she has poor vision and needs to lip-read.
- Try to minimize background noise (e.g., television sets, radio music) that can distract her from hearing you.
- When dining out, pick a quiet section of a restaurant to minimize background noise.
- At public shows and auditoriums, check to see if they have assisted listening devices you can get for her to use.
- At health care appointments, have health providers write down their recommendations for your mother to refer to if she has any doubt about what was said.

Sometimes we may feel embarrassed asking health providers to repeat something that was said. However, if a question remains unclear about how your mother should be caring for her health, you need to speak up and clarify what was said. Health care providers will appreciate your taking the time to clarify the treatment plans, as it helps ensure that their clients will be able to carry out the plan at home.

How can I help? If you notice someone is having problems hearing, encourage her to have her hearing checked.

Q. How will I know when I've been successful in helping someone with diabetes?

A. There are many ways to know you're effective as a helper. You may get a simple smile, a hug, or a heartfelt thank you. He may share with you how his diabetes management is going and report where his glycosylated hemoglobin (HbA1c) level is. These are all ways that signal a positive relationship. However, don't forget that the biggest compliment he gives you, as a helper, is when he confides his concerns and feelings to you. That he values your relationship and trusts you to the point of sharing his thoughts is something to feel proud and good about.

Q. I am so amazed at how healthful my friend who has diabetes eats. She always seems to have her weight under control. Is it possible for someone without diabetes to get on a diet like hers?

A. Yes. Because the diet for diabetes is simply a well-balanced meal plan and includes foods that are healthy for everyone to eat, there is no reason why friends and family members can't follow it, too!

To help you control your weight, you'll want to talk with a registered dietitian to review how you're currently eating and to create an individualized meal plan that fits your lifestyle and food preferences. If you let your friend know you'd like to follow a diet like hers, I'm sure she would be happy to help support you in your efforts and feel honored that you admire her healthy lifestyle habits.

Don't forget . . .   *positive relationships occur when people and friends can help each other. By showing your support and admiration of her efforts to stay healthy, you'll receive the benefits of a close relationship where she feels comfortable helping you in return. People helping people . . . that's what helps makes relationships strong and our world an enjoyable place to live in.*

Suggested Reading List

General Books

American Diabetes Association Complete Guide to Diabetes. American Diabetes Association, 1997.

Changing for Good. Prochaska, J. O., et al. Avon, 1994.

Diabetes A to Z: What You Need to Know About Diabetes—Simply Put, 3rd ed. American Diabetes Association, 1997.

Heartmates: A Guide for the Spouse and Family of the Heart Patient. Levin, R. F. Minerva Press, 1994.

Johns Hopkins Guide to Diabetes for Today and Tomorrow. Saudek, C. D., Rubin, R. R., and Shump, C. S. Johns Hopkins University Press, 1997.

Managing Type II Diabetes—Your Invitation to a Healthier Lifestyle, rev. ed. Monk, A., et al. Chronimed Pub, 1996.

Mars and Venus: Together Forever. Gray, J. HarperPaperbacks, 1994.

Raising a Child with Diabetes. Siminerio, J., and Betschart, J. American Diabetes Association, 1995.

Uncomplicated Guide to Diabetes Complications. Levin, M. E., and Pfeiffer, M. A., eds. American Diabetes Association, 1998.

When Diabetes Hits Home: The Whole Family's Guide to Emotional Health. Rapaport, W. S. American Diabetes Association, 1998.

Cookbooks

Cookbooks with Menu Planners

Magic Menus for People with Diabetes. American Diabetes Association, 1996.

Month of Meals. American Diabetes Association, 1998.

Quick and Healthy Meals

Art of Cooking for the Diabetic. 3rd ed. Hess, M. A. Contemporary Books, 1998.

Complete Quick & Hearty Diabetic Cookbook. American Diabetes Association, 1998.

Complete Step-by-Step Diabetic Cookbook. 3rd ed. Registered Dietitians from the University of Alabama at Birmingham. Oxmoor House, 1995.

Convenience Foods Cookbook. Cooper, N. IDC Publishing, 1998.

Diabetic Low-Fat, and No-Fat Meals in Minutes. Smith, M. J. Chronimed Publishing, 1996.

How to Cook for People with Diabetes. American Diabetes Association, 1996.

Quick & Healthy Recipes and Ideas, Vol. I & II. Ponichtera, B. American Diabetes Association, 1994, 1995.

Vegetarian Cooking for Healthy People. Meer, M. R., and Galeana, J. G. Appletree Press, 1997.

Desserts and Snacks

Diabetic Dessert Cookbook. Howard, C. and Seberg, G. H. Avon Books, 1997.

Joy of Snacks, rev. ed. Cooper, N. Chronimed Publishing, 1991.

Skinny Chocolate, Magida, P. and Grunes, B. Surrey Books, 1994.

Holiday and Ethnic Recipes

Flavorful Seasons Cookbook. Webb, R. American Diabetes Association, 1996.

Memorable Menus Made Easy. Webb, R. American Diabetes Association, 1997.

World-Class Diabetic Cooking—Great-Tasting Recipes from Around the World. Spicer, K. American Diabetes Association, 1996.

Associations/Agencies to Explore and Contact

Adaptive Environments Center, Inc., 374 Congress Street, Suite 301, Boston, MA 02210, 617/695-1225, (TDD), http://www.adaptenv.org

American Association of Diabetes Educators (AADE), 444 North Michigan Avenue, Suite 1240, Chicago, IL 60611-3901, 800/338-3633 or 312/644-2233, http://www.aadenet.org

American Diabetes Association, National Office, 1660 Duke Street, Alexandria, VA 22314, 800/232-3472, www.diabetes.org

American Dietetic Association, 216 West Jackson Blvd., Suite 800, Chicago, IL 60606-6995, 800/877-1600, http://www.eatright.org; Consumer Nutrition Hotline, 800/366-1655

Ask NOAH About: Diabetes Website, http://www.noah.cuny.edu/diabetes /diabetes.html

Association for Worksite Health Promotion, 60 Revere Drive, Suite 500, Northbrook, IL, 60062, 847/480-9574, http://www.awhp.org

Children with Diabetes, 5689 Chancery Place, Hamilton, OH 45011, 513/755-0186, http://www.childrenwithdiabetes.com

Disability Rights Education and Defense Fund, Inc., ADA Technical Assistance Hotline, 2212 Sixth Street, Berkeley, CA 94710, 510/644-2555 (TDD), http://www.dredf.org

Juvenile Diabetes Foundation International, 120 Wall Street, 19th floor, New York, NY 10005, 800/JDF-CURE or 212/785-9595, http://www.jdfcure.org

National Diabetes Information Clearinghouse, 1 Information Way, Bethesda, MD 20892-3560, 301/654-3327, http://www.niddk.nih. gov/health/diabetes/ndic.htm

National Information Center for Children and Youth with Disabilities, P.O. Box 1492, Washington, DC 20013, 800/695-0285

National Institute of Diabetes and Digestive and Kidney Diseases (NIDDK), *National Institutes of Health (NIH)*, Office of Communications and Public Liaison, NIDDK, NIH, 31 Center Drive, MSC 2560 Bethesda, MD 20892-2560, http://www.niddk.nih.gov

Rick Mendosa's Diabetes Directory, http://www.mendosa.com/diabetes. htm

U.S. Department of Justice: Americans with Disabilities Act Information Line, 800/514-0301 or 800/514-0383 (TDD), http://www.usdoj. gov/crt/ada/publicat.htm

U.S. Equal Employment Opportunity Commission, 1801 L Street, NW, Washington, D.C. 20507, 800/669-4000 or 800/669-6820 (TDD), http://www.eeoc.gov

Sample Menus

Sample Menu #1: Weekend Meals

Breakfast

Hot or cold cereal
Bagels, toasted
½ banana or grapefruit
Low-fat milk
Light margarine or cream cheese
Coffee or tea

Lunch

Tortilla wrap sandwich made from 1 tortilla stuffed with 2–3 oz. sliced deli meat, fresh vegetables, mustard or a teaspoon of mayonnaise (light)
Baked tortilla chips
Salsa
Fresh fruit slices
Low-fat milk or a sugar-free soft drink

Supper

3 oz. roast pork, grilled or baked
Rice (white, wild, or brown)
Steamed vegetables
Fresh bread or dinner roll
Salad made with mixed, fresh greens, optional
Angel food cake with fresh berries
Salad dressing and margarine (light)
Coffee or low-fat milk

Bedtime snack

Crackers and cheese

Sample Menu #2: Holiday Meals

Breakfast

Pancakes or waffles
Sausage links (if fat and sodium don't have to be restricted)
Fresh fruit or applesauce
Sugar-free or light syrup
Light margarine
Coffee or low-fat milk

Lunch

Turkey, roasted or grilled
Rice pilaf, stuffing, or mashed potatoes
Warm dinner rolls or fresh bread
Steamed vegetables
Assorted salad greens
Fruit salad or cranberry relish
Light margarine
Low-fat milk or tea

Supper

Lasagna (meat, cheese, or vegetable)
Tossed salad with assorted vegetables
Toasted garlic bread
Light salad dressing
Low-fat milk or coffee

Bedtime snack

Pretzels or popcorn

Sample Menu #3:
Light Meals

Breakfast
Corn flakes
Fresh fruit, sliced
English muffin, toasted
Peanut butter (optional)
Low-fat milk, coffee, or tea

Lunch
Low-fat cottage cheese salad with
   assorted fresh fruit slices
Vegetable soup
Fresh bread, tortilla, matzo, or
   crackers
Light margarine
Low-fat milk or sugar-free
   lemonade

Supper
Meat loaf with mushrooms
Potatoes, mashed or boiled
Steamed baby carrots
Warm dinner rolls or tortilla
Light margarine, optional
Sugar-free gelatin salad topped
   with fruit and a dollop of
   whipped topping
Low-fat milk or coffee

Bedtime Snack
Fresh fruit

References

Chapter 1

Adams, P. F., et al. "Current estimates from the National Health Interview Survey, 1994." National Center for Health Statistics. *Vital Health Stat* 10(193): 81–82, 1995.

American Diabetes Association. *Complete Guide to Diabetes*, 1997.

American Diabetes Association. *Diabetes Facts and Figures*, 1997. Online @http://www.diabetes.org.

American Diabetes Association. Economic consequences of diabetes mellitus in the US in 1997. *Diabetes Care* 21(2): 296–309, 1998.

American Diabetes Association. *Medical Management of Type 1 Diabetes*, 1998.

American Diabetes Association. *Medical Management of Type 2 Diabetes*, 1998.

American Diabetes Association. Who benefits from tight control and who doesn't. *Diabetes Advisor* 12(2): 12, 1998.

Bernstein, G. Medical tests explained: A guide to routine lab work. *Diabetes Self-Management* 15(2): 6–13, 1998.

Brewer, K. W., et al. Slicing the pie: Correlating HbA1c values with average blood glucose values in pie chart form. *Diabetes Care* 21(2): 209–212, 1998.

Carey, V. J., et al. Body fat distribution and risk of non-insulin-dependent diabetes mellitus in women. *Am J Epidemiology*, 145(7): 614–619, 1997.

Carter, J. S., et al. Non-insulin-dependent diabetes mellitus in minorities in the United States. *Annals of Internal Medicine* 125(3): 221–231, 1996.

Centers for Disease Control and Prevention. *Diabetes Surveillance*, 1997. Atlanta, GA: U.S. Department of Health and Human Services, 1997.

Centers for Disease Control and Prevention. *National Diabetes Fact Sheet: National estimates and general information in the United States.* Atlanta, GA: U.S. Department of Health and Human Services, Centers for Disease Control and Prevention, 1997.

Chan, J. C. N., et al. Diabetes in the Chinese population and its implications for health care. *Diabetes Care* 20(11): 1785–1790, 1997.

Cost effectiveness analysis of improved blood pressure control in hypertensive patients with type 2 diabetes: UKPDS 40. *British Medical Journal* 317(7160): 720–726, 1998.

Coustan, D. Gestational Diabetes Mellitus in: *Therapy for Diabetes and Related Disorders*, 3rd ed, 1998.

DeFronzo, R. A. Pathogenesis of type 2 diabetes: Metabolic and molecular implications for identifying diabetes genes. *Diabetes Reviews* 5(3) 177–269, 1997.

Diabetes Control and Complications Trial Research Group. The effect of intensive treatment of diabetes on the development and progression of long-term complications in insulin-dependent diabetes mellitus. *N Engl. J Med* 329(14): 977–986, 1993.

Dinsmoor, R. Beyond Type 1 and Type 2. *JDF International Countdown* pp. 26–29, Fall 1998.

Eisenbarth, G. Genetic counseling for Type 1 Diabetes in: *Therapy for Diabetes and Related Disorders*, 3rd ed, 1998.

Expert Committee on the Diagnosis and Classification of Diabetes Mellitus. Report of the Expert Committee on the Diagnosis and Classification of Diabetes Mellitus. *Diabetes Care.* 22(1): 55–19, 1999.

Fava, D., et al. Evidence that the age diagnosis of IDDM is genetically determined. *Diabetes Care* 21(6): 925–929, 1998.

Funell, M. M., ed. *Core Curriculum for Diabetes Education*, 3rd ed, 1998.

Gee, S. AGEing process. *Diabetes Forecast* 51(10): 72(3), 1998.

Harris, M., et al. Onset of NIDDM occurs at least 4–7 years before clinical diagnosis. *Diabetes Care* 15(7): 815, 1992.

Harris, M. I. NIDDM: Epidemiology and the scope of the problem. *Diabetes Spectrum* 9(1): 26–29, 1996.

Jeu, L., et al. Debunking the top diabetes myths. *Diabetes Self-Management* 15(5): 598–599, 1998.

King, H., et al. Global burden of diabetes: prevalence, numerical estimates, and projections, 1995–2025. *Diabetes Care* 21(9): 1414–1438, 1998.

Kissebah, A. H. Central obesity: measurement and metabolic effects. Diabetes Reviews 5(l): 8-20, 1997.

Levin, M. E., Pfeiffer, M.A., ed. *Uncomplicated Guide to Diabetes Complications*, 1998.

Maillet, N. A., et al. Using focus groups to characterize the health benefits and practices of black women with non-insulin-dependent diabetes. *Diabetes Educ* 22(1): 39–46, 1996.

Mayo Foundation. Diabetes medical essay. *Mayo Clinic Health Letter,* 1998.

McKenzie, S. B., et al. A primary intervention program (pilot study) for Mexican American children at risk for type 2 diabetes. *Diabetes Educ* 24(2): 180–187, 1998.

Muir, A., et al. *Endocrinol Metab Clin North Am* 21 (2): 201, 1992.

National Diabetes Information Clearinghouse. *Diabetes Control and Complications Trial* (DCCT), NIH Pub. No. 94-3874, 1992.

National Institute of Diabetes and Kidney Disease. *Diabetes Overview*, 1995.

National Institutes of Health. *Diabetes in America*, 2nd ed, Pub. No. 95-1468, 1995.

Perlmuter, L., et al. Does cognitive function decline in type II diabetes? *Diabetes Spectrum* 10(1): 57–62, 1997.

Peyrot, M. F., et al. Stress buffering and glycemic control: The role of coping styles. *Diabetes Care* 15(7): 842–846, 1992.

Rankin, S. H., et al. Quality of life and social environment as reported by Chinese immigrants with non-insulin-dependent diabetes mellitus. *Diabetes Educ* 23(2): 171–177, 1997.

Reece, E. A., et al. Management of Pregnant Women with Diabetes in: *Therapy for Diabetes and Related Disorders*, 3rd ed, 1998.

Rodeen, L. M., et al. New treatments for patients with diabetes. *Diabetes Spectrum* 11(1): 18–25, 1998.

Rosenbloom, A. L., et al. Non-insulin dependent diabetes mellitus (NIDDM) in minority youth: Research priorities and needs (NIDDM in Minority Children). *Clinical Pediatrics* 37(2): 143–153, 1998.

Saudek, C. D., et al. Implantable insulin pump vs multiple-dose insulin for non-insulin-dependent diabetes mellitus: a randomized clinical trial. JAMA 276(16)1322–1327, 1996.

Saudek, C. D., et al. *Johns Hopkins Guide to Diabetes for Today and Tomorrow*, 1997.

Tight blood pressure control and risk of macrovascular and microvascular complications in type 2 diabetes: UKPDS 38. *British Medical Journal* 317(7160): 703–713, 1998.

Trends in the prevalence and incidence of self-reported diabetes mellitus—United States, 1980–1994. *JAMA* 278(19): 1564–1565, 1997.

Trends in the prevalence and incidence of self-reported diabetes mellitus—United States, 1980–1994. *Morbidity and Mortality Weekly Report* 46(43): 1014–18, Oct. 31, 1997.

Zinman, B. Guidelines for the management of type 2 diabetes. In Olfesky, J.M. ed., *Current Approaches to the Management of Type 2 Diabetes: A Practical Monograph*, pp. 19–22, 1997.

Chapter 2

American Diabetes Association. Hypoglycemia: Beating the odds. *Diabetes Advisor*, 12: 22, 1998.

American Diabetes Association. *Complete Guide to Diabetes*, 1997.

Brown, S. A., et al. Symptom-related self-care of Mexican Americans with type 2 diabetes: Preliminary findings of the Starr County diabetes education study. *Diabetes Educ* 24(3): 331–339, 1998.

Coustan, D. Gestational Diabetes Mellitus in: *Therapy for Diabetes and Related Disorders*, 3rd ed, 1998.

Drass, J. A., et al. Knowledge about hypoglycemia in young women with type I diabetes and their supportive others. *Diabetes Educ* 21(1): 34–38, 1996.

Funell, M. M., ed. *Core Curriculum for Diabetes Education*, 3rd ed, 1998.

Gonder-Frederick, L., et al. The psychosocial impact of severe hypoglycemic episodes on spouses of patients with IDDM. *Diabetes Care* 20(10): 1543–1546, 1997.

Maynard, T. Exercise: Part I. Physiological response to exercise diabetes mellitus. *Diabetes Educ* 17(3): 196–205, 1991.

Nelson, J. K., ed. *Mayo Clinic Diet Manual: A Handbook of Nutrition Practices*, 7th ed, 1994.

Perlmuter, L. C., et al. Does cognitive function decline in type II diabetes? *Diab Spectrum* 10(l): 57–62, 1997.

Rajaram, S. S. Experience of hypoglycemia among insulin dependent diabetes and its impact on the family. *Sociol Health Illn* 19(3): 281–296, 1997.

Saudek, C. D., et al. *Johns Hopkins Guide to Diabetes for Today and Tomorrow*, 1997.

Weinger, K., et al. Blood glucose estimation and symptoms during hyperglycemia and hypoglycemia in patients with insulin dependent diabetes. *Am J Med* 98:22–31, 1995.

Chapter 3

American Diabetes Association. Nutrition recommendations and principles for people with diabetes mellitus: position statement. *Diabetes Care* 22(1): 542–545, 1999.

American Diabetes Association. Translation of the diabetes nutrition recommendations for health care institutions: Position statement. *Diabetes Care* 20(l): 106–108, 1997.

American Dietetic Association. *Nutrition Practice Guidelines for Type I and Type I Diabetes Mellitus*, 1996.

American Dietetic and Diabetes Association. *Exchange Lists for Meal Planning*, 1995.

Betty Crocker Kitchen Helper. Conimar Corporation, 1998.

Brown, S. L. Motivational strategies used by dietitians to counsel individuals with diabetes. *Diab Educ* 24(3): 313–318, 1998.

Darling, J. D., ed. *Better Homes and Gardens New Cook Book.* Meredith Books: Des Moines, IA, 1996.

Davis, D., et al. Food obstacles in intensive diabetes therapy. *Diabetes Spectrum* 11(l): 37-42, 1998.

Delahanty, L. M. Clinical significance of medical nutrition therapy in achieving diabetes outcomes and the importance of the process. *J Am Diet Assoc* 98(1): 28–30, 1998.

Ellwood, K. C. Methods available to estimate the energy values of sugar alcohols. *American Journal of Clinical Nutrition* 62(5): 1169, 1995.

Expert Committee on the Diagnosis and Classification of Diabetes Mellitus. Report of the Expert Committee on the Diagnosis and Classification of Diabetes Mellitus. *Diabetes Care* 22(1): S5–S19, 1999.

Franz, M. J. *Exchanges for All Occasions*, 4th ed., 1997.

Funell, M. M., ed. *Core Curriculum for Diabetes Education*, 3rd ed, 1998.

Garg, A. Management of dyslipidemia in IDDM patients. *Diabetes Care* 17(3): 224–234, 1994.

Gillespie, S. J. A carbohydrate is a carbohydrate is a carbohydrate: Is the ban on sugar really lifted? *Diabetes Educ* 22(5): 449, 451–2, 457, 1996.

Gillespie, S. Implementing liberalized carbohydrate guidelines: nutrition free-for-all or a more rational approach to carbohydrate consumption? *Diabetes Spectrum.* 9(3): 165-166. 1996.

Heilbronn, L. K., et al. Effect of energy restriction, weight loss, and diet composition on plasma lipids and glucose in patients with type 2 diabetes. *Diabetes Care.* 22(6): 889-895, 1999.

Holler, H. J., Pastors, J. G. *Diabetes Medical Nutrition Therapy: a Professional Guide to Management and Nutrition Education Resources*, 1997.

Kurtzweil, P. The new food label: coping with diabetes. *FDA Consumer,* 28(9): 20–25, November 1994.

Kurtzweil, P. New food label: making it easier to shed pounds. *FDA Consumer,* 28(6): 10–15, 1994.

Medications and supplements may trigger diarrhea. *Environmental Nutrition* 18(1): 3, 1995.

Monk, A., et al. *Managing Type I Diabetes: Your Invitation to a Healthier Lifestyle*, 1996.

Nelson, J. K., ed. *Mayo Clinic Diet Manual: A Handbook of Nutrition Practices*, 7th ed, 1994.

Payne, M. L. Sorbitol is a possible risk factor for diarrhea in young children. *Journal of the American Dietetic Association*, 97(5): 532–534., 1997.

Powers, M. A., ed. *Handbook of Diabetes Medical Nutrition Therapy*, 2nd ed., 1996.

Rombaurer, I. S., et al. *All New, All Purpose, Joy of Cooking*. Scribner: New York, NY 1997.

Schafer, R. G., et al. Translation of the diabetes nutrition recommendations for health care instututions. *Diabetes Care* 20(1): 96–105, 1997.

Schlundt, D, et al. Situational obstacles to dietary adherence for adults with diabetes. *J Am Diet Assoc.* 94(8): 874-879, 1994.

Stehlin, D. A *Little 'Lite' Reading*, @ http://www.fda.gov/fdac/special/foodlabel/lite.html , 1998.

U.S. Department of Agriculture. *Nutrition and Your Health: Dietary Guidelines for Americans*, 4th ed., 1995.

Warshaw, H. *Diabetes Meal Planning Made Easy: How to Put Food Pyramid to Work for Your Busy Lifestyle*, 1996.

Chapter 4

American Diabetes Association. Complete Guide to Diabetes, 1997.

Becton-Dickinson. Answers to questions about sick days. Getting Started. 1998

Coustan, D. *Therapy for Diabetes and Related Disorders,* 3rd ed, p. 21, 1998.

Cypress, M., et al. Hunting down the hazards of hypoglycemia. *Diabetes Self-Management* 9(1): 10–16, 1992.

Davis, D., et al. Food obstacles in intensive diabetes therapy. *Diabetes Spectrum* 11(1): 37–42, 1998.

Funell, M. M., ed. *Core Curriculum for Diabetes Education,* 3rd ed, 1998.

Gori, M., et al. Pharmacy update: Natural products and diabetes treatment. *Diabetes Educ* 24(2): 201–208, 1997.

Gori, M., et al. Pharmacy update: Sugar-free medications. *Diabetes Educ* 23(3): 269–278, 1997.

HealthPartners. *Diabetes and Sick Day Care,* 1996.

Kelley, D. B. *Medical Management of Type 2 Diabetes,* 4th ed, 1998.

Saudek, C. D., et al. *Johns Hopkins Guide to Diabetes for Today and Tomorrow,* 1997.

Chapter 5

Becton-Dickinson. *Planning Your Diabetes Care . . . During Disaster Conditions,* 1997.

Dendinger, M. J. Traveling with diabetes: Business as usual. *Diabetes Self-Management* 15(3): 7–13, 1998.

Dunning, D. Safe travel tips for the diabetic patient. *RN* April: 51–54. 1989.

Hope Heart Institute. *During the Holidays . . . How Not to Get Stuffed.*

Chapter 6

Adams, P. F., et al. *National Center for Health Statistics: Current Estimates from the National Health Interview Survey,* 1991, Vital Statistics Series 10(184), 1993.

American Diabetes Association. Economic consequences of diabetes mellitus in the US in 1997. *Diab Care,* 21(2): 296–309, 1998.

American Diabetes Association. Here's what you thought. *Diabetes Forecast* 48(3): 56–58, 1995.

Burton, W. N. Evaluation of a Worksite-Based Patient Education Intervention Targeted at Employees with Diabetes Mellitus *JOEM* 40:702–706, 1998.

Carter, M. New medical law with help seniors pay for supplies and education. *Diabetes Forecast* 51(8): 43–45, 1998.

Centers for Disease Control and Prevention. *Diabetes Surveillance,* 1997, U.S. Dept of Health and Human Services, 1997.

Congressional Budget Office. *Preliminary Cost Estimate for the Medicare Preventive Benefits Improvement Act,* 1996

Freedman, E. The changing world of disability management. *Managing Employee Health Benefits* 6(4): 41–45, 1998.

Goetzel, R. Z., et al. Health care costs of worksite health promotion participants and non-participants. *JOEM* 40(4): 341–346, 1998.

Goetzel, R. Z., et al. The relationship between modifiable health risks and health care expenditures. *JOEM* 40(10): 843–854, 1998.

Heins, J. M., et al. The Americans with disabilities act and diabetes. *Diabetes Care* 17(5): 453, 1994.

Hoffman, C., et al. Persons with chronic conditions: Their prevalence and costs. *JAMA* 176: 1473–1479, 1996.

Lloyd, C. E., et al. Education and employment experiences in young adults with type 1 diabetes mellitus. *Diabetic Med* 9:661–666, 1992.

Mas, F. S., et al. Hispanics and worksite health promotion: Review of the past, demands for the future. *J Community Health* 22(5): 361–371, 1997.

McNeil, J. M. *Americans with Disabilities: 1991–92*, U.S. Bureau of the Census Current Population Report, P70–33, 1993.

Padgett, D. L., et al. Employers' perceptions of diabetes in the workplace. *Diabetes Spectrum* 8(1): 10–15, 1995.

Padgett, D. L., et al. Managing diabetes in the workplace: Critical factors. *Diabetes Spectrum* 9(1): 13–20, 1996.

Papenfuss, R. L. Worksite health promotion and disease prevention. *Prim Care* 21:387–390, 1994.

Ratner, R. E. Working around employment discrimination. *Diabetes Self-Management* 9(1): 33–35, 1992.

Rice, D. P., La Plante, M. P. Medical expenditures for disability and disabling comorbidities. *Am J. Public Health* 82: 739–471, 1992.

Robinson, N., et al. Employment problems and diabetes. *Diabetes Medicine* 7:16–22, 1990.

Rumrill, P. D., Millington, M. J., Webb, J. M., Cook, B. G. Employment expectations as a differential indicator of attitudes toward people with insulin-dependent diabetes mellitus. *Journal of Vocational Rehabilitation* 10(3): 271–280, 1998.

Songer, T. The influence of diabetes on the social and economic events of men. *Diabetes Spectrum* 11(2): 93–100, 1998.

Songer, T. J. Disability in diabetes. In *Diabetes in America*, 2nd ed., 1995.

Songer, T. J., et al. Employment spectrum of IDDM. *Diabetes Care* 12:615–22, 1989.

Testa, M. A., Simonson, D.C. Health economic benefits and quality of life during improved glycemic control in patients with type 2 diabetes mellitus. *JAMA* 280(17): 1490–1496, 1998.

Tobin, C. T. Getting the most from managed care. *Diabetes Self-Management* 15(4): 21–28, 1998.

U.S. Department of Health and Human Services, Public Health Service. *National Survey of Worksite Health Promotion Activities: Summary Report,* 1993.

U.S. Equal Employment Opportunity Commission—Enforcement Statistics. *Americans with Disabilities Act of 1990 (ADA) Charges FY 1991–FY 1997,* online @ http://www.eeoc.gov, 12/14/98.

U.S. Department of Justice. *Americans with Disabilities Act Handbook,* online @ http://www.usdoj.gov/crt/ada/adahom1.htm, 12/14/98.

Vogt, T. M., et al. The medical care system and prevention: The need for a new paradigm. *Medical Care System and Prevention* 12(1): 5–13, 1998.

Walsh, P. Good company. *Diabetes Forecast* 49(9): 44–47, 1996.

Chapter 7

American Diabetes Association. *Diabetes Info: Beating Bad Feelings,* online @ http://www.diabetes.org, 10/30/97.

American Diabetes Association. More from spouses. *Diabetes Forecast* 50(8): 49–58, 1997.

American Diabetes Association. Spouses speak out. *Diabetes Forecast* 50(7): 70–72, 1997.

Anderson K., et al. (ed), *Mosby's Medical, Nursing, and Allied Dictionary,* 1997.

Baum, N. Treating impotence. *Diabetes Self-Management* 15(6): 37–47, 1998.

Bee, H. L. *Journey of Adulthood,* 1987.

Breitrose, P. E. Stress, anger, and depression: How emotions affect your risk of a heart attack. *Diabetes Self-Management* 15(4): 7–10, 1998.

Carey, M. P., et al. Reliability and validity of the appraisal of diabetes scale. *J Behav Med* 14(1): 43–51, 1991.

D/ART. *Depressive Illnesses Are a Major Public Health Problem,* online @ http://www.nimh.nih.gov/dart, 12/11/98.

DCCT Research Group. Reliability and validity of a diabetes quality-of-life measure for the diabetes control and complications trial (DCCT). *Diabetes Care* 11(9): 725–732, 1988.

De Veciana, M. Diabetes and female sexuality. *Diabetes Reviews* 6(l): 54–64, 1998.

Ellison, G. C., et al. Exemplar's experience of self-managing type 2 diabetes. *Diabetes Educ* 24(3): 325–330, 1998.

Faulk, J. S. Coping with complications. *Diabetes Self-Management* 15(2): 70–73, 1998.

Finston, P. Quitting the self-blame game. *Diabetes Forecast* 46(12): 46–49, 1993.

Flower, J. The skills of the change master. *Physician Exec* 22(11): 34–36, 1996.

Gabriel, Y. Psychoanalytical contributions to the study of the emotional life of organizations. *Administration & Society* 30(3): 291–314, 1998.

Gasbarro, R. Antidepressants: How not to live with depression. *Diabetes Self-Management* 15(3): 43–48, 1998.

Goleman, D. *Emotional Intelligence*, 1995.

Grey, M., et al. Short-term effects of coping skills training as adjunct to intensive therapy in adolescents. *Diabetes Care* 21(6): 902–908, 1998.

Hendricks, L. E., et al. Greatest fears of type 1 and type 2 patients about having diabetes: Implications for diabetes educators. *Diabetes Educ* 24(2): 168–173, 1998.

Kelley, D. B. *Medical Management of Type 1 Diabetes*, 3rd ed, 1998.

Lamberg, P. J. Treating depression in medical conditions may improve quality of life. *JAMA* 276(11): 857–858, 1996.

Levin, R. F. *Heartmates®: A Guide for the Spouse and Family of the Heart Patient*, 1994.

Levine, S. B., Fones, C. Psychological aspects at the interface of diabetes and erectile dysfunction. *Diabetes Reviews* 6(l): 41–49,1998.

Lundman, B., et al. Coping strategies in people with insulin-dependent diabetes mellitus. *Diabetes Educ* 19(3): 198–204, 1993.

Lustman, P. J., et al. Identifying depression in adults with diabetes. *Clinical Diabetes* 15: 78–81, 1997.

Lustman, P. J., et al. Treatment of major depression in adults with diabetes: A primary care perspective. *Clinical Diabetes* 15(3): 122–128, 1997.

Marrero D. G., et al. Fear of hypoglycemia in the parents of children and adolescents with diabetes: maladaptive or healthy response? *Diab Educ*, 23(3): 281–286, 1997.

Mazur, M. L. The best support system in the world. *Diabetes Forecast* 50(7): 20–26, 1997.

Morley, J. E. Sex hormones and diabetes. *Diabetes Reviews* 6(l): 6–15, 1998.

Okun, B. F. *Effective Helping: Interviewing and Counseling Techniques*, 5th ed, 1997.

Phillipson, S. Coping with sexual dysfunction. *Diabetes Self-Management* 15(6): 32–36, 1998.

Pollin, I. Coping with diabetes: Don't let the winds of change knock you off your feet. *Diabetes Forecast* 49(5): 24–28, 1996.

Polonsky, W. H. *Emotional Intelligence: A Seminar for Health Professionals*, presented 11/5/98 in Minneapolis, MN.

Riebe, D., et al. Setting the stage for healthy living. *ASCM's Health & Fitness Journal* 2(3): 11–15, 1998.

Ruge, K. Dealing with the diagnosis: Where do you go from here? *Diabetes Self-Management* 15(3): 49–52, 1998.

Seid, R. P. The agonies and the ecstasies: The truth about emotions. *Shape* 16(6): 100–106, 1997.

Seligman, M. E. P. What you can change & what you cannot change. *Psychology Today* 27(3): 34–46, 1994.

Strong, M. *Mainstay: For the Well Spouse of the Chronically Ill*, 3rd ed, 1997.

Taibbi, R. Taking control: Putting the brakes on self-destructive behaviors. *Diabetes Self-Management* 15(5): 76–81, 1998.

Wahba, A. F. Caring and … curing. *RN* 57(5): 39–40, 1994.

Chapter 8

American Diabetes Association. Diabetes mellitus and exercise. *Diabetes Care* 22(1): S49–S53, 1999.

Anderson, R. M., et al. Using focus groups to identify diabetes care and education issues for Latinos with diabetes. *Diabetes Educ* 24(5): 618–625, 1998.

Anderson, R. M., et al. Using focus groups to psychosocial issues of urban black individuals with diabetes. *Diabetes Educ* 22(1): 28–33, 1996.

Ashworth, P. Breakthrough or bandwagon? Are interventions tailored to stage of change more effective than non-staged interventions? *Health Education Journal*, 56:166–174, 1997.

Berg, B. R. One thing you can count on: Your life will always change. *Diabetes in the News* 13(2): 40–41, 1994.

Buxton, K., et al. How applicable is the stages of change model to exercise behavior? A review. *Health Ed J* 55: 239–257, 1996.

Cardena, L., et al. Adult onset DM: Glycemic control and family function. *Am J Sci Med* (293): 28–33, 1987.

Carey, M. P., et al. Reliability and validity of the appraisal of diabetes scale. *J Behav Med* 14(1): 43–51, 1991.

CDC Health Communication Evaluation Services. Draft: Health eating and physical activity: Focus group research with contemplators and pre-parers. Task 08: Formative Research for a National Nutrition and Physical Activity Health Communication Campaign, Center for Disease Control and Prevention, July 1995.

CDC Health Communication Evaluation Services. Draft: Health eating and physical activity: Concept testing focus group research. Task 927608: Formative Research for a National Nutrition and Physical Activity Health Communication Campaign, Center for Disease Control and Prevention, January 1996.

Corey, M. S., et al. *Becoming a Helper*, 1989.

Covey, S. R. *The 7 Habits of Highly Effective People: Powerful Lessons in Personal Change*, 1990.

DCCT Research Group. Reliability and validity of a diabetes quality-of-life measure for the diabetes control and complications trial (DCCT). *Diabetes Care* 11(9): 725–732, 1988.

Fisher, L., et al. Family and type 2 diabetes: A framework for intervention. *Diabetes Educ* 24(5): 599–607, 1998.

Griffith, L. S., et al. Depression in women with diabetes. *Diabetes Spectrum* 10(3): 216–225, 1997.

Konen, J. C., et al. Family function, stress and locus of control: Relationships to glycemia in adults with diabetes mellitus. *Arch Family Med* 1993 (2): 393–402, 1993.

Lipton, R. B., et al. Attitudes and issues in treating Latino patients with type 2 diabetes: Views of healthcare providers. *Diabetes Educ* 24(1): 67–71, 1998.

McGinnis, A. L. *Bringing Out the Best in People*, 1985.

Meillier, L. K., et al. Reactions to health education among men. *Health Educ Res* I 1 (1): 107–115, 1996.

Peyrot, M. F., et al. Stress buffering and glycemic control: The role of coping styles. *Diabetes Care* 15(7): 842–846, 1992.

Polonsky, W. H., et al. Listening to our patients' concerns: Understanding and addressing diabetes-specific emotional distress. *Diabetes Spectrum* 9(1): 8–11, 1996.

Prochaska, J. O., et al. *Changing for Good*, 1994.

Prochaska, J. O., et al. In search of how people change: Applications to addictive behaviors. *American Psychologist* 47(9): 1102–1114, 1992.

Prochaska J. O., Velicer, W. F. The transtheoretical model of behavior change. *Am J Health Promotion* 12(l): 38-43, 1997.

Rollnick, S., et al. Methods of helping patients with behavior change. *British Med J* 307(6897): 188–191, 1993.

Sandoval, W. Stages of change: a model for nutrition counseling. *Top Clin Nutr* 9(3): 64–69, 1994.

Schafer, L. C., et al. Supportive and nonsupportive family behaviors: Relationship to adherence and metabolic control in persons with type 1 diabetes. *Diabetes Care* 9(9): 179–185, 1986.

Sigman-Grant, M. Stages of change: A framework for nutrition interventions. *Nutr Today*, 31(4): 162–171,1996.

Stott, N. C. H., et al. Limits to health promotion: They lie in individual's readiness to change. *Br Med J* 309(6960): 971–972, 1994.

Sullivan, E. D., et al. Struggling with behavior changes: A special case for clients with diabetes. *Diabetes Educ* 24(1): 72–74, 1998.

Swift, C. S., et al. Attitudes and beliefs about exercise among persons with non-insulin-dependent diabetes. *Diabetes Educ* 21(6): 533–540, 1995.

Trief, P. M., et al. Family environment, glycemic control, and the psychosocial adaptation of adults with diabetes. *Diabetes Care* 21(2): 241–245, 1998.

Tufts University. The six stages of change. *Tufts University Diet and Nutrition Letter* 14: 5, 1996.

Verity, L. S., et al. Getting fit with fits and starts. *Diabetes Forecast* 51(9): 74–78, 1998.

Chapter 9

American Diabetes Association. Sabotage! Are your loved ones guilty? *Diabetes Advisor* 12(5): 15, 1998.

Bradley, C. *Handbook of Psychology and Diabetes*, rev. ed., 1994.

Bustanoby, A. Making your mate your best friend. *Marriage* 24(4): 12–15, 1994.

Chalmers, K., et al. Should you be eating that? *Diabetes Educ* 20(1): 66–69, 1994.

Corey, M. S., et al. *Becoming a Helper*, 1989.

Fitzgerald, J. T., et al. Gender differences in diabetes attitudes and adherence. *Diabetes Educ* 21(6): 523–529, 1995.

Gray, J. *Mars and Venus: Together Forever*, rev. ed, 1994.

Kelsey, K., et al. Is social support beneficial for dietary change? A review of the literature. *Fam Community Health* 20(3): 70–82, 1997.

Konen, J. C., et al. Family function, stress, and locus of control. *Arch Fam Med* 2: 393–402, 1993.

McGinnis, A. L. *Friendship Factor*, 1979.

Mengel, M. B., et al. The relationship of family dynamics/social support to patient functioning in IDDM patients on intensive insulin therapy. *Diab Research Clinical Practice* 9:149–1162, 1990.

Okun, B. F. *Effective Helping: Interviewing and Counseling Techniques*, 5th ed, 1997.

Palardy N., et al. Adolescents' Health Attitudes and Adherence to Treatment for Insulin-Dependent Diabetes Mellitus. *J Dev Behav Pediatr* 19:31–37, 1998.

Polonsky, W. H. Besieged by the diabetes police. *Diabetes Self-Management* 12(5): 21–26, 1995.

Polonsky, W. H. Blowing away the holiday blues. *Diabetes Self-Management*, 11(6): 42–48, 1994.

Rubin, R. R., et al. Men and diabetes: Psychosocial and behavioral issues. *Diabetes Spectrum* 11(2): 81–87, 1998.

Ruge, K. Surviving diabetes as a couple. *Diabetes Self-Management* 14(5): 28–35, 1997.

Sturkie, J., et al. *Peer Helper's Pocketbook*, 1992.

Trief, P. M., et al. Family environment, glycemic control, and the psychosocial adaptation of adults with diabetes. *Diabetes Care* 21(2): 241–245, 1998.

Index

A

advanced glycation end products (AGEs), 43
alcoholic beverages, 110–11
ALT approach, 249–52
associations and agencies, 259–60

B

balanced menus, 85–87, 89
blood glucose levels, 9, 15, 90, 114–34. *See also* glucose
fluctuating levels, 26–27
blood pressure, 42
blood testing, 20. *See also* tests for diabetes
borderline diabetes, 16–17
brittle diabetes, 25–26

C

calcium, 100–102
carbohydrate counting, 93–94
carbohydrates, 52, 53, 83, 106–8
low carbohydrate diets, 107–8
treating hypoglycemia, 51–53
care during illness, 114–34. *See also* flu; illnesses
causes of diabetes, 11–14
Centers for Disease Control (CDC), 38, 161–62
change, stages of, 225–30
cholesterol, 41, 94–97

combination foods, 87–88
communication, 175–178, 234–255
complications, 35–36, 38–41
autonomic neuropathy, 41
dental disease, 39
eye disease, 33–34, 39
heart disease, 39
high blood pressure, 39
hypoglycemic unawareness, 158
kidney disease, 39
nerve problems, 40–41
neuropathy, 40–41
control, 31, 63, 66–67, 181–83
cookbooks, 88, 257–58
cooking tips, 94–102, 109, 113. *See also* meals
coping with emotions, 190–219. *See also* emotions
coworkers, 154–60. *See also* work environments

D

dental disease, 39
depression, 196, 212–13
diabetes, 5–45
borderline, 16–17
brittle, 25–26
causes of, 11–14
complications, 35–36, 38–41

diabetes *(continued)*
  definition of, 7
  diagnosis, 15–16
  facts, 5–45
  gestational (GDM), 10, 14, 16, 43–44
  heart disease, 94
  idiopathic, 13
  insulin-dependent diabetes mellitus (IDDM). *See* type 1 diabetes
  maturity-onset diabetes of the young (MODY), 11
  myths, 32–37, 103–9
  non-insulin dependent-diabetes mellitus (NIDDM). *See* type 2 diabetes
  past treatment, 6–7, 25–26, 31
  pattern management, 27
  pills, 20–21
  risk assessment, 44–45
  symptoms, 18–19
  tests for, 15–16, 24–25, 41–43. *See also* tests for diabetes
  treatment, 19–21. *See also* treating diabetes
  type 1, 9–10. *See also* type 1 diabetes
  type 2, 10. *See also* type 2 diabetes
  types of, 9–11, 30–31
Diabetes Control and Complications Trial (DCCT), 35–36, 102
diabetic diet, 75–80
diabetic foods, 108–9, 111–12. *See also* foods; meals
diabetic ketoacidosis (DKA), 116–18
  symptoms, 117–18

diabetiquette, 187–88
diet, healthy, 225, 234–35, 256. *See also* healthy habits; meals
disability, 160–62, 164–65
disclosing illness, 156–60, 164–65
discrimination, 156, 162–68
doctor appointments, 218–19, 254–55
  being truthful, 218–19
  understanding doctor's directions, 254–55

E
eating away from home, 148–49, 209
eating habits, 240–41, 244
emotions, 190–219
  acceptance, 145–46, 196, 198
  anger, 196, 222–23, 252–54
  ambivalence, 145–46, 221
  bargaining, 196
  caring for others, 203–5
  coping methods, 200
  coping skills, 195–202
  coping strategies, 202, 224–25
  denial, 196
  depression, 196, 211–13
  excuses, 64–65, 210, 219
  expressing, 193–95
  fear at night, 70–71, 218
  feeling overwhelmed, 197–98
  first reactions, 190–93, 195–96
  frustration, 207–10, 219, 236, 254
  grief, 195–96
  guilt, 206–7
  helping others, 207–9, 222–23, 234–35, 255
  helplessness, 203–5

moodiness, 59–62, 211–13
nagging, 213–14, 225–27,
    232–33, 236
negativity, 198–99
purpose of, 193–95
quiz on caring, 205
quiz on coping, 199–200
quiz on feelings, 191–93
shock, 195
worry, 148–50, 203–5, 211,
    213–17, 219
etiquette, 187–88
exchange lists, 89–92
    sick-day foods, 126
    starches, 91
exercise, 64–65, 241, 244–45
eye dilation, 42
eye disease, 39

F
finger-stick blood glucose test,
    24–25
first reactions, 5, 195–96
flu, 120–28. *See also* illnesses
    meals for sick days, 121–28,
        130
    sick-day meal plan, 122, 125
    sick friends and neighbors,
        131–34
Food Guide Pyramid, 83–86, 90
food labels, 95, 104–7, 111
foods, 76–78. *See also* healthy
    habits; meals
    avoid, 76–80
    combination foods, 87–88
    diabetic, 108–9, 111–12
    for guests with diabetes,
        72–73, 80–81, 109–10
    free foods, 92–93
    high-fat foods, 94–97

low-fat foods, 94–97
    sick-day foods, 124–27
    snacks, 152–53
    special occasions, 135–39
    stomach upset, 112, 127
    sugar substitutes, 112–13
foot inspection, 42–43
fructosamine, 41
fructose, 103, 107
fruit, 103

G
genetics, 12–14
gestational diabetes, 10, 14–16,
    43–44
    causes of, 14
gifts for those with diabetes,
    131–34
glucagon, 54–56
    definition of, 55–56
    injections, 55–56
    kits, 55–56
glucose, 7–8, 26–27
    above normal, 7, 15–17,
        26–27
    control, 63, 66–67, 181–83
    definition of, 7–8
    factors affecting, 27
    high blood glucose, 114–34
    impairment, 18
    levels, 57–59, 233
    low blood glucose, 46–71
    meters, 24–26
    normal levels, 9
    patterns, 27
    tests, 15
glycogen, 7
glycosylated albumin, 41
glycosylated hemoglobin
    (HbA1c), 41, 42, 43

golden rules, 57, 123
guests with diabetes, 72–73, 80–81, 109–10

H

habits, changing, 220–30. *See also* healthy habits
  five stages, 225–30
  recognizing stages, 228–30
healthy eating, 82–83
healthy habits, 220–36, 256
  avoid nagging, 224, 225, 233, 236
  blood glucose levels, 233
  changing habits, 220–24, 225–27, 230–34
  do's and don'ts, 232
  family's habits, 221
  following diet, 225, 234–35
  motivation, 225, 230–32
  proactive thinking, 223–24
  promoting health, 221–22
  reactive thinking, 223–24
  stages of change, 225–30
  support, 231–32, 239–47, 255
hearing loss, 254–55
heart disease, 39, 94
helping others, 207–9, 239–43, 245–47, 253–56
hemoglobin A1. *See* glycosylated hemoglobin
herbs, 36–37, 99–100
high blood glucose, 114–34. *See also* hyperglycemia
high blood pressure, 39, 97–100
honeymoon phase, 31
hyperglycemia, 115–16
  causes of, 115
  dangers, 115–16
  definition of, 115

diabetic ketoacidosis (DKA), 116–19
hyperglycemic hyperosmolar non-ketotic syndrome (HHNS), 118–19
  ketones, 116–19
  symptoms, 118
hypoglycemia, 47, 51–53, 67–71
  15/15 rule, 51–53, 56–57
  blood glucose control, 63, 66–67
  blood glucose levels, 57–59
  carbohydrates, 53
  causes of, 47
  definition of, 46
  do's and don'ts, 54–55
  emergency guidelines, 54–55, 179–80
  hypoglycemic unawareness, 58–59
  insulin reaction, 46, 60–62
  mood changes, 59–60
  pregnancy, 68–69
  symptoms, 47–50
  testing, 50–51
  treatment, 50–55, 66–67
  while sleeping, 70–71, 218
hypoglycemic unawareness, 58

I

idiopathic diabetes, 13
illnesses, 120–34
  cough drops, 128–29
  flu, 120–21
  helping sick friends and neighbors, 131–34
  hospital stay, 129
  loss of appetite, 127–28
  meals for sick days, 121–28, 130

impaired fasting glucose (IFG),
　18
impaired glucose tolerance
　(IGT), 18
impotence, 217
insulin, 20–24
　definition of, 7, 24
　injections, 22–23, 28
　pumps, 28–29
　reaction, 46. *See also* insulin
　　reaction
　shock, 46
　types of, 21–23
insulin-dependent diabetes
　mellitus (IDDM). *See* type 1
　diabetes
insulin reaction, 46, 64–65
　glucagon, 62
　in school, 69–70
　treating, 60–62
　while sleeping, 70–71, 218
insulin shock, 46

J
job-related issues, 154–89. *See
　also* work environments

K
ketones, 116–19
　tests for, 119
kidney disease, 39, 100–102

L
lipid, 41
listening skills, 176, 247-52
　ALT approach, 249–52
living alone with diabetes, 214–17
　checking in, 214–17
　emergency plans, 215
　visual checkpoints, 216–17

low blood glucose, 46–71. *See
　also* hypoglycemia
low-fat cooking tips, 94–97

M
maturity-onset diabetes of the
　young (MODY), 11
meals, 72–113. *See also* healthy
　habits
　alcoholic beverages, 110–11
　balanced meals, 85–87
　calcium, 100–102
　carbohydrate counting, 93–94
　combination foods, 87–88
　diabetic desserts, 108–9,
　　111–12
　diabetic diet, 75–77
　diabetic foods, 108–9
　dietetic, 105–6
　exchange lists, 89–92, 126
　Food Guide Pyramid, 83–86,
　　90
　food labels, 95, 104–7
　foods to avoid, 76–80
　for guests with diabetes,
　　72–73, 80–81, 109–10
　free foods, 92–93
　fruit, 103
　high-fat foods, 94–97
　high-protein, 106–8
　low-carbohydrate, 106–8
　low-fat foods, 94–97
　low-sodium, 97–100
　meat, 100–102
　nutrition myths, 102–9
　nutrition quiz, 73–74
　portion sizes, 79
　potassium, 100–102
　sample menus, 88–89, 91,
　　261–62

meals *(continued)*
  sick days, 121–28, 130
  skipping, 77
  special occasions, 135–39,
    184–87
  spices, 99–100
  stomach upset, 112, 127
  sugar, 104–5
  sugar, forms of, 107
  sugar-free, 105–6
  sugar substitutes, 112–13
  taste, 103–4
  well-balanced, 83–87
medical insurance, 173–75
menus, sample, 88–89, 91,
    261–62. *See also* meals
mood changes, 59–60,
    211–13
motivation, 230–32
myths, 32–37, 102–9

N
nagging, 213–14, 224–25, 233,
    236
nerve problems, 40–41
neuropathy, 40–41
  autonomic, 41
  peripheral, 40
nighttime low, 70–71, 218
non-insulin-dependent-diabetes
    mellitus (NIDDM), 10
normal blood glucose level, 9
nutrition, 73. *See also* healthy
    habits
  myths, 102–9
  quiz, 73–74

O
oral glucose tolerance test
    (OGTT), 15

P
pancreas, 7, 8, 21
pancreatic disorders, 14
pills for diabetes, 20–21
potassium, 100–102
pregnancy, 68–69
proactive thinking, 223–24

R
reactive thinking, 223–24
relationships, 237–56
  communication skills, 239,
    245, 248–52
  eating habits, 244
  exercise habits, 244–45
  friends, 237–39, 256
  helping others, 245–47,
    253–56
  listening skills, 176, 247–48,
    249–52
  positive, 237–38
  retaining independence,
    253–54
  self-awareness quiz, 240–46
  support, 238–39

S
school environment, 188–89
  Disabilities Education Act,
    188–89
  Rehabilitation Act of 1973,
    188–89
  testing blood glucose levels,
    189
  treating hypoglycemia, 189
sexual concerns, 65, 217
skipping meals, 77
snacks, 152–53
sodium, 97–100
sorbitol, 107, 112

special occasions, 135–53. *See also* meals
  anniversaries, 146–47
  birthdays, 147, 185
  conferences, 151–52, 186–87
  gatherings, 151–53
  gifts for those with diabetes, 131–34
  holiday meals, 135–39, 143–46
  holiday traditions, 144–45
  meetings, 151–52
  school, 70
  stress-free holidays, 139–43
  vacations, 148–50
  visits, 80–81, 109–11, 150–51
  weddings, 147–48
stomach upset, 112, 127
stress, 137–39
sugar, 104–5
  forms of, 107
  non-calorie sweeteners, 113
  substitutes, 112–13
  treating hypoglycemia, 66–67
sweeteners, 113
symptoms, 18–19, 47–50, 49, 117–18

T

tests for diabetes, 15–16, 20, 41–43
  blood glucose, 15
  blood pressure, 42
  eye dilation, 42
  finger-stick blood glucose, 24–25
  foot inspection, 42–43
  glycosylated albumin, 41
  glycosylated hemoglobin (HbA1c), 41
  HbA1c levels, 42
  lipid panel, 41
  oral glucose tolerance test (OGTT), 15
  urine analysis, 42
  urine glucose, 119–20
traveling, 67–68, 148–50
treating diabetes, 19–20
  blood testing, 20
  healthful eating, 19–20
  insulin, 20
  lifestyle habits, 20
  pills, 20
type 1 diabetes, 9–10, 20
  causes of, 11–12
  environmental factors, 12
  genetics, 12–13
  idiopathic diabetes, 13
  immune response, 11–12
  risk factors, 45
  viral factors, 12
type 2 diabetes, 9–10, 17, 20, 30–31
  age, 13
  causes of, 13–14
  environmental factors, 13–14
  genetics, 13
  lifestyle, 13
  obesity, 13
  risk factors, 44, 45
  self-assessment quiz, 44

U

United Kingdom Prospective Diabetes Study (UKPDS), 35–36, 102
urine analysis, 42
urine glucose tests, 119–20

V

viral factors, 12

W

weight loss, 106–8
work environments, 154–89
  Americans with Disabilities
    Act, 156, 161, 163, 164–65,
    166
  blood glucose control, 181–83
  Centers for Disease Control
    (CDC), 161–62
  coaching, 175–78, 181–82
  communication, 177–78
  coworkers, 154–60
  diabetes-friendly, 170–73
  disabilities, 160–62
  disclosing illnesses, 156–60,
    164–65, 177–78, 183–84

  discrimination, 156, 162–68
  emergency plan, 179–81
  employees, 175–78
  Equal Employment
    Opportunities Commission,
    165
  etiquette, 187–88
  fairness, 166–70, 175–77
  injections, 183–84
  insulin reaction, 177–78,
    180–81
  lunch, 185–87
  lunch meetings, 186–87
  medical insurance, 173–75
  schools, 188–89
  special occasions, 184–85
  special treatment, 169–70
  supporting employees,
    175–77